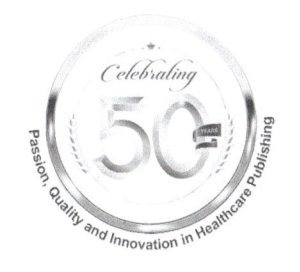

Medical X-ray Film Processing

Medical X-ray Film Processing

Second Edition

K Thayalan
MSc DipRP PhD DSc FUICC FIMSA FUSI FICRO
Consultant Medical Physicist and Head
Medical Physics Division
Dr Kamakshi Memorial Hospital Pvt Ltd, Chennai
Ex-Professor
Barnard Institute of Radiology and Oncology
Madras Medical College
Chennai, Tamil Nadu, India

Foreword
Prof **C Amarnath**

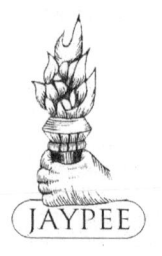

WN
150
.T373
2021

JAYPEE BROTHERS MEDICAL PUBLISHERS
The Health Sciences Publisher
New Delhi | London

Jaypee Brothers Medical Publishers (P) Ltd

Headquarters
Jaypee Brothers Medical Publishers (P) Ltd
4838/24, Ansari Road, Daryaganj
New Delhi 110 002, India
Phone: +91-11-43574357
Fax: +91-11-43574314
E-mail: jaypee@jaypeebrothers.com

Overseas Office
JP Medical Ltd
83 Victoria Street, London
SW1H 0HW (UK)
Phone: +44 20 3170 8910
Fax: +44 (0)20 3008 6180
E-mail: info@jpmedpub.com

Website: www.jaypeebrothers.com
Website: www.jaypeedigital.com

© 2021, Jaypee Brothers Medical Publishers

The views and opinions expressed in this book are solely those of the original contributor(s)/author(s) and do not necessarily represent those of editor(s) of the book.

All rights reserved. No part of this publication may be reproduced, stored or transmitted in any form or by any means, electronic, mechanical, photocopying, recording or otherwise, without the prior permission in writing of the publishers.

All brand names and product names used in this book are trade names, service marks, trademarks or registered trademarks of their respective owners. The publisher is not associated with any product or vendor mentioned in this book.

Medical knowledge and practice change constantly. This book is designed to provide accurate, authoritative information about the subject matter in question. However, readers are advised to check the most current information available on procedures included and check information from the manufacturer of each product to be administered, to verify the recommended dose, formula, method and duration of administration, adverse effects and contraindications. It is the responsibility of the practitioner to take all appropriate safety precautions. Neither the publisher nor the author(s)/editor(s) assume any liability for any injury and/or damage to persons or property arising from or related to use of material in this book.

This book is sold on the understanding that the publisher is not engaged in providing professional medical services. If such advice or services are required, the services of a competent medical professional should be sought.

Every effort has been made where necessary to contact holders of copyright to obtain permission to reproduce copyright material. If any have been inadvertently overlooked, the publisher will be pleased to make the necessary arrangements at the first opportunity. The **CD/DVD-ROM** (if any) provided in the sealed envelope with this book is complimentary and free of cost. **Not meant for sale.**

Inquiries for bulk sales may be solicited at: jaypee@jaypeebrothers.com

Medical X-ray Film Processing

First Edition: **2005**

Second Edition: **2021**

ISBN: 978-93-89587-92-0

Printed at Repro India Limited

Dedicated to

My late mother Mrs Arukkani

and

Late father Mr K Kuppusamy

Foreword

*"We lose ourselves in books,
we find ourselves there too"*

It gives me immense pleasure to write the foreword for this book on *Medical X-ray Film Processing* written by my beloved teacher and renowned Physicist, Prof K Thayalan. I have known him since my postgraduate student days in Madras Medical College and I have always been fascinated by his understanding of Radiology physics as a subject.

Eventhough he has written over six books on basic radiological physics, this book is unique in its approach to both conventional and digital X-rays, comparing and contrasting the physics behind both equipments.

In this digital era, the understanding of fundamental concepts about Darkroom and conventional X-ray film processing is important for technicians working in rural hospitals and isolated hospitals/clinics. This book with its crystal clear concepts will guide the technicians and definitely promote simple, safe and economical Diagnostic Radiology.

This book, like all his other books will help the BSc and RIT Radiology students in learning about X-rays and medical X-ray films through its simple language and line diagrams. Also, it will come in handy during examinations for postgraduate medical students.

"To teach is to touch a life forever"

May Prof K Thayalan continue to teach and enrich the lives of technicians and students across the country through his books and I wish him all the best in all his future endeavours.

Prof C Amarnath
Head, Department of Radiodiagnosis
Government Stanley Medical College
Chennai, Tamil Nadu, India

Preface to the Second Edition

I am happy and proud to write this second preface after fifteen years. The first edition came in 2005 and lot of developments have taken place over the years in X-ray film processing. Originally, the book dealt with basics of Medical X-ray films, which are used to record X-ray images as hard copy. The impact of X-rays is so much that, no patient goes without X-ray in some form or other. Off late, the use of X-ray film (screen-film) is reduced and computed radiography and digital radiography have occupied its place in a phased manner. Still X-ray films and dark rooms are partly used in many hospitals. There is a need to understand the screen-film technology and digital radiography systems. Even in digital radiography, special films are being used to record the final image as hard copy.

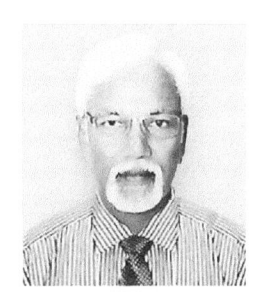

Attempts are being made to incorporate all the above new modalities, their basics, work flow, technical details, etc., in a systematic manner. This second edition consists of 10 chapters, which are tailored to the present needs, by incorporating recent developments. Screen-film radiography, digital radiography, their image quality, artifacts and quality assurance are discussed in detail. Attempts are made to include fundamental concepts, production of X-rays and radiological health and safety, to suit the undergraduate syllabus of radiography and imaging technology course. To explain the principles in an easy way, figures and tables are used wherever required.

I look forward to your healthy comments and suggestions.

K Thayalan

Preface to the First Edition

Medical X-ray film plays a vital role in diagnostic imaging. It is the final hard copy obtained in each investigation or examination. The film becomes the document/property of the hospital or patient and decides many critical issues. Improper storage and inadequate processing certainly will weaken the image quality. Hence, proper understanding of X-ray film and its environment is very much essential.

The various steps involved in making the final hard copy, shall be carried out in organized and optimal way. The persons handling the film processing, and the student community must be educated sufficiently, so that well-trained manpower may be generated, in this country.

I hope that this book may provide useful information that is required in the above field. Probably this is the first book of this nature, addressing various relevant topics collectively. I thank M/s Jaypee Brothers Medical Publishers (P) Ltd, New Delhi, India for undertaking this publication.

I dedicate this book to my late father Mr K Kuppusamy. Healthy comments and suggestions are invited from the readers.

K Thayalan

Acknowledgements

I am thankful to my wife T Tamilselvi, son T Parthiban and daughter T Kayal Vizhi for their love, support and cooperation.

I acknowledge Dr Kamakshi Memorial Hospital Pvt Ltd. and the Managing Director, and my medical physics colleagues, especially Ms X Sidonia Valas, Ms S Purnima, and Mr T Godwin Paul Das for their assistance and support during the book writing process. I thank Prof C Amarnath, Head, Department of Radiodiagnosis, Government Stanley Medical College, Chennai, Tamil Nadu for having written the foreword for this book.

I am also thankful to Shri Jitendar P Vij (Group Chairman), Mr Ankit Vij (Managing Director), Ms Chetna Malhotra Vohra (Associate Director—Content Strategy), Ms Pooja Bhandari (Production Head) of M/s Jaypee Brothers Medical Publishers (P) Ltd, New Delhi, India, for publishing this book as usual, in neat and elegant manner.

Contents

1. **Fundamental Concepts** 1
   - Units and Measurements *1*
   - Force, Work, Power, and Energy *1*
   - Temperature and Heat *4*
   - Electric Charge, Potential, and Current *5*
   - Atoms and Molecules *6*
   - Electromagnetic Radiation *9*
   - Photography *12*
   - Flexible Film *14*

2. **Production of X-rays** 20
   - Discovery of X-rays *20*
   - Modern X-ray Tube *24*
   - Interaction of Radiation with Matter *33*
   - Radiation Quantities and Units *36*
   - X-ray Images *38*

3. **Medical X-ray Film** 39
   - Film Structure *39*
   - Film Technology *42*
   - Film Type, Size, and Packing *45*
   - Characteristics of X-ray Film *51*
   - Film Handling and Storage *54*

4. **Darkroom, Cassette, and Intensifying Screens** 56
   - Darkroom *56*
   - Cassette *62*
   - Intensifying Screens *64*

5. **X-ray Film Processing** 74
   - Manual X-ray Film Processing *74*
   - Preparation of the Baths *81*
   - Influence of Time and Temperature *82*
   - Replenisher *83*
   - Automatic Film Processor *84*
   - Solutions for Automatic Processor *89*
   - Multiformat Imaging *93*
   - Chemical Pollution *96*

xvi Medical X-ray Film Processing

6. Screen-film Image Quality, Artifacts and Quality Assurance..................97
   - Image Quality 97
   - Artifacts 113
   - Quality Assurance 113

7. Digital Radiography 123
   - Digital Systems 123
   - Computed Radiography 127
   - Charged-coupled Devices 134
   - Digital Radiography Systems 136

8. Digital Radiography; Image Quality, Viewing, and Recording 146
   - Image Quality 146
   - Digital Image Viewing 154
   - Recording of Digital Image 161
   - Picture Archiving and Communication System 166
   - Optimal Image Quality in Digital Radiography 168

9. Digital Radiography; Image Artifacts and Quality Assurance............. 170
   - Image Artifacts 170
   - Digital Radiography Artifacts 170
   - Computed Radiography Artifacts 178
   - Image Compression 182
   - Quality Control 183

10. Radiological Health and Safety 193
    - Biological Effects of Radiation 193
    - System of Radiation Protection 196
    - Methods of Radiation Control 198
    - Regulatory Requirements in the use of X-ray Equipment 201
    - Responsibilities of Employer, Licensee, Radiological Safety Officer (RSO) and Radiation Workers 204
    - Personnel Monitoring Systems 208

Bibliography 213

Index 215

1

Fundamental Concepts

UNITS AND MEASUREMENTS

Physics is a science dealing with nature. It is very important to study the properties of material bodies in nature, under different physical conditions. Measurements of physical quantity such as length, mass, and time are essential to understand the properties of material bodies. Any physical quantity is measured accurately only in terms of a standard of its own kind. The standards which are defined and accepted by all are called the units. For example, distance is measured in meter, mass in kilogram and time in seconds.

System International

The System International (SI) has seven fundamental units as given below:
- Length: meter (m)
- Mass: kilogram (kg)
- Time: second (s)
- Electric current: ampere (A)
- Temperature: kelvin (K)
- Luminous intensity: candela (cd)
- Amount of substance: mole (mol)

Units of Length, Mass, and Time

Meter: One meter is the length equal to 16,50,763.73 wavelengths of the orange-red light emitted by the individual atoms of krypton – 86, in a krypton discharge lamp kept at 15°C and 76 cm of mercury.

Kilogram: One kilogram is equal to the mass of the platinum-iridium alloy cylinder (prototype) of diameter equal to its height kept at the International Bureau of Weights and Measures at Serves, near Paris, France.

Time: The second is defined as the duration of 9,19,26,31,770 periods of the radiation corresponding to the unperturbed transition between two specified energy levels of the ground state of cesium-133 atom.

FORCE, WORK, POWER, AND ENERGY

Matter may be defined as that which occupies space and affects our senses continually. A limited portion of our matter is called material body. A material body may be considered to be made up of very large number of particles.

Motion and Speed

A body is said to be in motion, if it changes its position continuously with respect to its surroundings. The speed of a body is the rate at which it describes its path. Here, the direction of motion is not taken into account. Thus, speed has only magnitude hence, it is a scalar quantity.

Displacement, Velocity, Acceleration, and Momentum

Displacement of a moving body is its change of position measured by a straight line joining the initial and final positions of the body. It has both magnitude and direction. The velocity of a moving body is the rate of change of displacement. The unit of velocity is m/s and it is a vector quantity. Acceleration of a moving body is its rate of change of its velocity. The unit of acceleration is m/s^2.

The acceleration exerted by the earth on the body is called the *acceleration due to gravity* of the earth. It is denoted by the letter g and the value of g varies from place to place. For practical calculations, the approximate value of g is 9.8 m/s^2. The *momentum* (P) of a moving body is the product of mass (m) and velocity (v) and it is given the relation:

$$P = mv$$

The momentum is a vector quantity and its direction is the same as its velocity, the unit is $kg.ms^{-1}$.

Inertia and Force

Newton has showed that all material bodies have inertia. It is the inability of any object to change itself its state of rest or of uniform motion. Force is the action exercised on a body, so that it changes the state of rest or of uniform motion of the body. It is measured by the product of mass (m) of the body and the acceleration (a) produced by the force on the body (F = ma). The SI unit of force is *newton* and it is denoted by the letter N. One newton is the force acting on a body of mass 1 kg, producing an acceleration of 1 m/s^2. There are four physical forces in the universe, namely *gravitational, electrostatic, strong* and *weak forces*.

Pressure

The total force acting on a liquid surface is called *thrust*. The pressure (p) is defined as the force (F) per unit area (A) and its unit is Nm^{-2} or *Pascal* (Pa). The atmospheric pressure is about 1.01×10^5 Pa. The pressure is caused by the weight of material pressing on its surface. It may be also due to collisions of atoms or molecules of a gas within a container. The pressure of a liquid at rest is always perpendicular to the surface in contact with it. The pressure at a point within a liquid is directly proportional to the depth of the point from the free surface, density, and acceleration due to gravity.

Fundamental Concepts

Scalar and Vector Quantities

All physical quantities can be classified into two broad categories namely, scalar and vector quantities. Quantities that have only magnitude and no direction are called scalar quantities, e.g. length, mass, time, etc. Quantities that have a magnitude as well as direction are called vector quantities, e.g. displacement, velocity, force, etc.

A vector quantity is usually represented by a line with an arrow head ($\rightarrow$). The magnitude of the vector is shown by the length of the line and the direction of the arrow represents the direction. To find the resultant of scalar quantities, they are simply added algebraically. To find the resultant of two or more vector quantities simple algebraic addition is not applicable. The addition of vector is done by the parallelogram law or the polygon law of vectors.

Mass and Weight

The mass of a body is the quantity of matter contained in it. It is measure of its resistance to acceleration. A weight of a body is the force of attraction exerted by the earth on it. If m is the mass of a body and g is the acceleration due to gravity at a given place, then weight = mg newtons.

Work

If a force acts on a body and the point of application of the force moves, then work is said to be done by the force. If the force F is applied and it moves the body through a distance s, in its direction then work done (W) = F × s. The unit of work is *joule* (J). One joule is the amount of work done when the point of application of a force of one newton moves a body through a distance of one meter.

Power

The rate of doing work (W) is called power. It is measured by the amount of work done in unit time (t). Power = W/t. The unit of power is *watt*. 1 watt = 1 J/s. One *horsepower* (HP) is equal to 750 W. The power consumed at the rate of one *kilowatt* for 1 hour is called 1 kilowatt-hour, which is = 36×10^5 J.

Energy

The energy of a body is its capacity to do work. It is measured by the amount of the work that it can perform. The unit of energy is joule. Usually, radiation energy is measured by the unit *electron volt* (eV). There are many forms of energy such as mechanical energy, heat energy, light energy, chemical energy, electrical energy, and atomic energy. There are two forms of mechanical energy, such as:
- Potential energy
- Kinetic energy

Potential energy of a body is the energy it possesses by virtue of its position. It is calculated by the relation mgh, where m is the mass of the body, g is the acceleration due to gravity and h is the height from the earth. The kinetic energy of a body is the energy possessed by it due to its motion. Kinetic energy = $mv^2/2$, where v is the velocity and m is the mass of the body. Energy can neither be created nor be destroyed, but can be transformed from one form to another. **Einstein** showed that mass and energy are interchangeable ($E = mC^2$), where E is the energy, m is the mass and C is the velocity of light. In diagnostic radiology, energy is measured in electron volt, which will be discussed later.

Density

The density of a body (ρ) is defined as the ratio of its mass (m) and volume (v) and its unit is kgm^{-3}. The density of a body is same, if it is made up of identical material. If its composition is changed, its density will vary.

$$\rho = m/v$$

The *relative density or specific gravity* of a substance is the ratio between its density and that of water.

Mole

The amount of matter in a body is expressed by the number of elementary particles (atoms or molecules) it contains and its unit is mole. One mole of matter contains 6.022×10^{23} elementary particles, and it is known as *Avogadro's number*.

TEMPERATURE AND HEAT

Every matter is made up of atoms and molecules. The atoms are always in movement and hence, possess kinetic energy. This kinetic energy is responsible for the hotness and coldness of a body. Temperature is the measure of hotness or coldness of a body. Temperature is measured in degrees with the help of thermometers. Temperature is measured either in *fahrenheit (°F) or celsius (°C) or in kelvin (K)*.

All thermometers have lower fixed point and upper fixed point. The temperature of melting point of ice is taken as the lower fixed point. The temperature of steam is taken as the upper fixed point. In the fahrenheit scale, the lower fixed point is 32 and the upper fixed point is 212. The interval between the two points is divided into 180 equal points. In the celsius scale the lower fixed point is 0 (zero) and the upper fixed point is 100. The interval between the two points is divided into 100 equal points. Zero degree centigrade (celsius) is equal to 273 kelvin. The relation between celsius and fahrenheit is given by $C/100 = (F - 32)/180$.

Heat is a form of energy which can be transformed from one place to another. There are three methods of heat transfer, namely *conduction*, *convection*, and *radiation*. The conduction and convection process require a medium, whereas the radiation process needs no medium for heat transfer. Heat is measured in joule or *calorie*. 1 calorie = 4.2 joules.

ELECTRIC CHARGE, POTENTIAL, AND CURRENT

Charge (Q)

The term electric is derived from the Greek word *electron*. Electric bodies are said to possess electric charge. There are two types of charges, namely;
○ Positive charge
○ Negative charge.

Two like charges repel each other and two unlike charges attract each other. Electric charge in nature comes in units of one magnitude (e) only. Hence, any body can have charges only in multiples of e. The charges can neither be created nor be destroyed. Materials which allow charges to pass through them are called conductors, e.g. metals, human body, earth, etc. Bodies which do not allow the charge to pass through are called insulators, e.g. glass, mica, plastic, etc. The unit of charge is *coulomb*. One coulomb is the charge which when placed at a distance of 1 m in air or vacuum from an equal and similar charge, experiences a repulsive force of 9×10^9 N. As per the revised definition, one coulomb is equal to the charge carried by 6×10^{18} electrons or protons. The electric charge of one electron is 1.6×10^{-19} C.

Potential (V)

The space around a charge in which its influence is felt is known as electric field. The electric potential at a point in an electric field is the work done in taking a unit positive charge from infinity to that point. The unit of potential is *volt*. The potential difference between two points is said to be 1 volt, if the work done in moving a unit charge from one point to other point is 1 J.

Current (I)

Application of voltage in an electrical circuit causes the electrons to move. The positive end is called anode and the negative end is called cathode. The flow of electric charge in a conductor is called an electric current. The direction of current is always opposite to the flow of electrons. It is defined as the rate of flow of charge through any section of a wire. The unit of current is *ampere* (A). The electric current through a wire is called one ampere, if one coulomb of charge flows through the wire in one second. Electric power is the product of current (I) and voltage (V). Electric power consumption is measured in kilowatt (kW). Power supply is provided either in single phase or three phase. The three phase power supply provides much more power than single phase. The frequency of alternating current in India is 50 cycles/second.

Ohm's Law

The Ohm's law states that a steady current flowing through a metallic conductor is proportional to the potential difference between its ends, provided the temperature remains constant. If I is the current in ampere and V is the potential difference in volts then, $I \propto V$, at constant temperature, i.e. $I = V/R$, where R is a constant known as the *resistance* of the conductor.

Resistance

Resistance is the property of a conductor by which it opposes the flow of current. It is defined as the ratio between the potential difference and current of the conductor, i.e. $R = V/I$. The device, which offers resistance to the flow of current, is called *resistor*. It is represented by zig-zag lines. The resistor with variable resistance is called *rheostat*.

The unit of resistance is *ohm* (Ω). The ohm is the resistance of the conductor through which a steady current of one ampere passes, when a potential difference of one volt exists across it.

ATOMS AND MOLECULES

Everything in the world is made up of one or more of the basic substance called elements, e.g. carbon, iron, mercury and oxygen. Elements consist of tiny bits of matter called atoms. An atom is defined as the smallest indivisible particle of an element that can take part in a chemical reaction. Atom can join together to form larger chemical units called molecule. For example, two atoms of hydrogen combine with one atom of oxygen and form the water molecule (H_2O). Thus, molecules are the smallest part of an element or a compound which exist in a free and separate state.

Nucleus

Scientific discoveries proved that the atoms contain still smaller particles such as *protons, neutrons and electrons* (Fig. 1.1). These particles are called subatomic particles. Proton is a positively charged particle, whereas the electron is a negatively charged particle. Neutron is electrically neutral

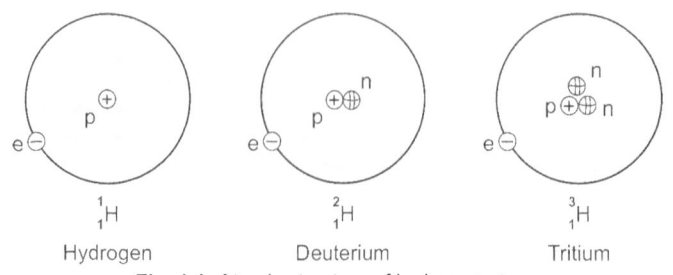

$${}^{1}_{1}H \quad\quad {}^{2}_{1}H \quad\quad {}^{3}_{1}H$$

Hydrogen   Deuterium   Tritium

Fig. 1.1: Atomic structure of hydrogen atom.

Fundamental Concepts

and has no charge. The protons and neutrons are clustered at the center of the atom, called nucleus. The protons and neutrons are called *nucleons*. The electrons are arranged outside the nucleus, which are orbiting in circular and elliptical paths. *Atomic mass unit (amu)* is the unit of mass in atomic scale.

Atomic Number and Mass Number

The number of protons in an atom is equal to the number of electrons. This is called the *atomic number (Z)*. The sum of the protons and the neutrons present in the nucleus of an atom is called the *mass number (A)*. Atoms with same atomic number but with different mass numbers are called *isotopes*. Isotopes with unstable nuclei, which are capable of performing radioactivity is called as *radioisotopes*. The electron has very little mass. The proton mass is roughly equal to that of 1,836 electrons. The mass and charge of these particles are given in Table 1.1.

Arrangement of Electrons

The electrons revolve around the nucleus in circular orbits corresponding to different energy levels. These energy levels are called shells, namely K, L, M, etc. Each shell is at a definite distance from the nucleus. The maximum number of electrons that can be accommodated in any shell can be found by the formula $2n^2$, where n is the number of the shell. Thus, K, L, and M shell can have 2, 8, and 18 electrons, respectively. The arrangement of electrons in different shells, for the first five elements is given in Table 1.2.

Table 1.1: The mass and charge of subatomic particles.

Particle	Mass, kg	Charge, Coulombs
Proton	1.66×10^{-27}	1.6×10^{-19}
Neutron	1.7×10^{-27}	Nil
Electron	1/1836 proton mass	-1.6×10^{-19}

Table 1.2: Arrangement of electrons in different shells.

Elements	Mass number	Atomic number	K	L	M
Hydrogen (H)	1	1	1	—	—
Helium (He)	4	2	2	—	—
Lithium (Li)	7	3	2	1	—
Beryllium (Be)	9	4	2	2	—
Boron (B)	11	5	2	3	—

No. of electrons in shells

Ionization

An atom is normally electrically neutral. If one or more orbital electrons are removed from the atom, the remainder of the atom is left with positively charged and is known as positive ion. This process of removal of orbital electrons from the neutral atom is known as ionization. Sometimes, one or more electrons may attach themselves to a neutral atom and form a negative ion. This is also known as ionization. Any radiation that have sufficient energy to eject atomic electron is called ionizing radiation, e.g. X-rays and gamma rays. Ionizing radiation is further divided into directly ionizing (e.g. electrons and protons) and indirectly ionizing radiations (e.g. neutrons, X-rays and gamma rays).

Binding Energy

To produce ionization, energy must be given to an orbital electron, in order to remove it from the atom. There is a force of attraction between the electron and the positively charged nucleus. Therefore, the energy which is just sufficient to remove an electron from the orbit is known as binding energy. The magnitude of the binding energy depends on the atomic number and the shell from which the electron is being removed. It is greater for elements of higher atomic number and greatest for the K shell (innermost shell). The K-shell binding energy increases with atomic number. The binding energy of the outer shell electron is small.

Binding energies are negative because they represent amounts of energy that must be supplied to remove electrons from atoms. Electron shells are often described in terms of the binding energy of electrons occupying the shells, e.g. the binding energy is –13.5 eV for an electron in the K shell and –3.4 eV for an electron in the L shell of hydrogen atom, respectively. The K-shell binding energies of various elements are given in Table 1.3. To remove a K-shell electron, one has to supply energy equal or greater than the binding energy of that K-shell electron.

Table 1.3: Atomic number (Z) and binding energies (E_k) of few elements.

Element	Z	E_k, keV
Aluminium	13	1.6
Calcium	20	4
Molybdenum	42	20
Iodine	53	33
Barium	56	37
Gadolinium	64	50
Tungsten	74	70
Lead	82	88

Excitation

In an atom, if energy is supplied, the electrons can be moved from the inner orbits to the outer orbits. Now the atom will have more energy than its normal state. It is said to be in an excited state and the process is known as excitation. For example, to move an electron from K to L shell of the hydrogen atom, the energy required is (−3.4 eV) − (−13.5 eV) = 10.1 eV. If there is a vacancy in the K-shell, it will be filled by an electron from a higher shell. The electron moving from the outer shell to inner shell may emit its excess energy in the form characteristic X-rays. Sometimes, the characteristic X-rays supply energy and remove orbital electrons. Such electrons removed from the same atom are called *Auger electrons*.

Electron Volt

When energy is measured in the macroscopic level, units such as joule and kilowatt-hour are used. In the microscopic level, the electron volt (eV) is a more convenient unit of energy. Hence, eV is used as the unit of energy in radiation physics. One eV is the kinetic energy imparted to an electron, accelerated across a potential difference of one volt.

$$1 \text{ eV} = 1.6 \times 10^{-19} \text{ J}$$
$$= 1.6 \times 10^{-12} \text{ erg}$$
$$= 4.4 \times 10^{-26} \text{ kWh}$$

The electron volt describes potential as well as kinetic energy. The binding energy of an electron in an atom is a form of potential energy. Kilo electron volt (keV) and million electron volt (MeV) are also used as units in practice.

$$1 \text{ keV} = 10^3 \text{ eV and}$$
$$1 \text{ MeV} = 10^6 \text{ eV}.$$

ELECTROMAGNETIC RADIATION

An electric charge is surrounded by an electric field. If the charge moves, a magnetic field is produced. When the charge undergoes an acceleration or deceleration, the magnetic and the electric fields of the charge will vary. The combined variation of the electric and magnetic fields result in loss of energy. The charge radiates this energy in a form known as electromagnetic radiation. The electromagnetic radiation moves in the form of sinusoidal waves (transverse waves) in a straight line (Fig. 1.2).

The electromagnetic wave possesses *wavelength* (λ), *frequency* (ν), *and velocity* (c). The distance between two consecutive positive peaks is known as wavelength. The number of cycles of the wave which passes a fixed point per second is known as the frequency of the wave. The velocity of the wave is the distance traveled per second by the wave. The relation between wavelength, frequency, and velocity of the electromagnetic wave can be expressed as $c = \nu\lambda$. All electromagnetic waves travel at

Medical X-ray Film Processing

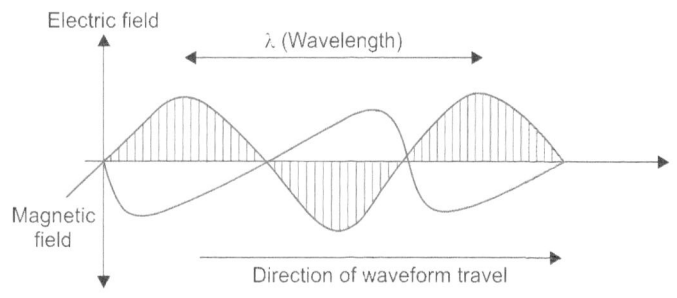

Fig. 1.2: Electromagnetic radiation.

the same velocity in a given medium. In vacuum, the velocity is about 2.998×10^8 m/s. Frequency is measured in cycles per second or hertz (Hz), and wavelength is measured in meter.

Quantum Nature of Radiation

Though electromagnetic radiation has the properties of waves, it also behaves like a stream of small bullets each carrying a certain amount of energy. This bundle of radiation energy is called a *quantum or photon*. The photon has no mass and behaves as wave or particle. The amount of energy carried by the photon depends upon the frequency of the radiation. The actual amount of energy (E) carried by a photon is given by the equation $E = h\nu$, where h is the *Planck's constant* equal to 6.63×10^{-34} Js. Substituting the value of $\nu = c/\lambda$ in the above equation, the energy is given by:

$$E = hc/\lambda = 124/\lambda$$

The product of the velocity of light (c) and Plank's constant (h) is 124. E is measured in keV and λ is in nanometers (nm). It is seen that the energy of the photon is inversely proportional to its wavelength. As the wavelength decreases, the energy increases. Low frequency radiation has long wavelength, whereas high frequency radiation has short wavelength.

Electromagnetic Spectrum

Electromagnetic spectrum includes radiation from very long radio waves to short penetrating gamma rays. All of them travel at a velocity c in a vacuum. The wavelength and photon energy of the whole range of electromagnetic radiations are summarized in Table 1.4. Radio waves have low frequency and gamma rays have high frequency. There is no physical difference between X-rays and gamma rays of same energy.

Luminescence

When electromagnetic radiation falls on certain crystalline substance, visible or ultraviolet light is emitted from the crystal. This phenomenon

Table 1.4: The wavelength and photon energy range of electromagnetic radiations.

Radiation	Wavelength	Frequency	Energy
Radio waves	1,000–0.1 m	0.3–3,000 MHz	0.001–10 µeV
Microwaves	100–1 mm	3–300 GHz	10–1,000 µeV
Infrared	100–1 µm	3–300 THz	10–1,000 meV
Visible light	700–400 nm	430–750 THz	1.8–3 eV
Ultraviolet	400–10 nm	750–30,000 THz	1.8–100 eV
X- and Gamma rays	1 nm–0.1 pm	3×10^5–3×10^9 THz	1 keV–10 MeV

is called luminescence. The material that emits light is called luminescent material or phosphor. Luminescence is similar to characteristic X-ray emission, but involves outer shell electron of the atom. When a luminescent material is exposed to X-rays, the outer shell electron of its atom is in the excited state. Thus, a vacancy is created in the outer shell and making the atom unstable. The above vacancy is filled when the excited electron returns to the normal state. During this transition, visible light is emitted. The excited energy and the wavelength emitted depend on the structure and character of the phosphor material.

There are two types of luminescence, namely (i) *fluorescence* and (ii) *phosphorescence*. Fluorescence is a form of light emission within 10^{-8} s of X-ray exposure. If the emission of light is delayed beyond 10^{-8} s, it is called phosphorescence. This means that whenever phosphor is exposed to X-rays, one can see fluorescence emission. If the X-ray exposure is stopped, fluorescence will cease. Whereas, in phosphorescence the phosphor continues to emit light even after the X-ray exposure ceases. Actually, the crystal absorbs the radiation of shorter wavelength which produces excitation in the crystal. Due to subsequent electronic transition, the crystal emits radiation of energy in the visible region, e.g. *zinc-cadmium sulfide and calcium tungstate*.

Inverse Square Law

The intensity of electromagnetic radiation is proportional to the number of photons crossing an unit area per second. The intensity decreases with distance in a non linear fashion. This non-linear fall off in intensity with distance is called inverse square law. Hence, the intensity of electromagnetic radiation is inversely proportional to the square of the distance from its source. Let us consider a point source s, emitting radiation at constant rate. The radiation spread over the inner surface of an imaginary sphere of radius d with surface area $4\pi d^2$. Then the radiation intensity at a point d is given by the relation;

$$I \propto \frac{1}{d^2}$$

12 Medical X-ray Film Processing

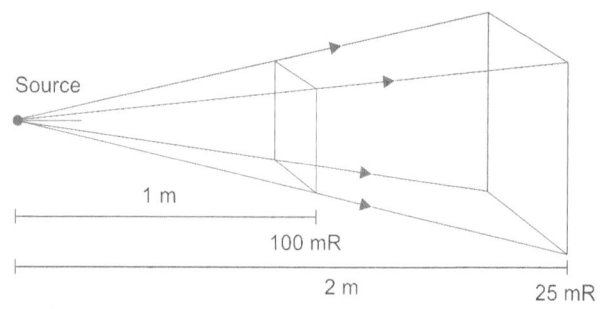

Fig. 1.3: Inverse square law: As the distance increases by 2, the radiation intensity decreases by a factor of 4.

If the distance is doubled, the intensity decreases by a factor of 4 (Fig. 1.3). The inverse square law is based on the following assumptions:
- The source of radiation is a point source
- The radiation travels in straight line
- The radiation is emitted equally in all directions
- The energy is radiated at a constant rate
- No radiation energy is lost on its way from the source to the point of measurement.

PHOTOGRAPHY

Photography is method of forming durable image by the action of light, which was invented by Joseph **Nicephore Niepce** in 1826. He exposed his plate by light for 8 hours, but the image was not sharp (Fig. 1.4). He used a portable camera *obscura* to expose a *pewter plate* coated with *bitumen* to light. Photography is a Greek word meaning drawing or writing (graphy) with light (Photo). The credit goes to Louis J.M. Daguerre (1839) for the establishment of chemical development of a photo sensitive material. He placed an exposed plate (silver salt fused with iodine) in the cupboard. Later date, he found a well defined positive image on the plate. There was some mercury spillage in the cupboard, and its fumes had developed the image. Niepce had collaboration with **Louis Daguerre** and created a new system *Daguerreotype*. It is a copper plate coated with silver and exposed to iodine vapor, before the exposure of light. It required a light exposure of about 15 min and become very popular at that time.

The credit goes to **William F. Talbot** (England, 1839) for inventing the negative-positive method of photography. He found that he could develop a latent image after the exposure of a silver halide to light. The name photography was coined by **Sir John Herschel** in 1839, while writing a letter to William F.Talbot. He also coined the words, negative and positive regarding photographic images.

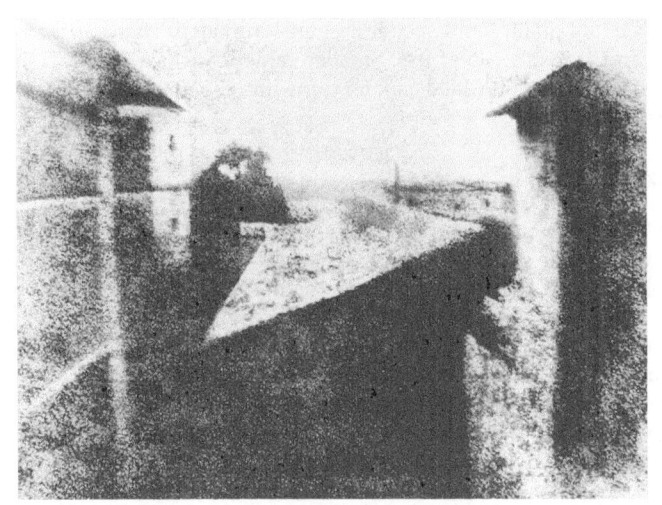

Fig. 1.4: First photograph of John Nicephore Niepce (1827) by using his camera Obscura.
(*Source*: Arthur G et al, Radiographics, 1989).

Emulsion Plates

Later, emulsion plates replaced the Daguerreotype, due to its lower cost and short exposure time in seconds. These plates are basically wet plates, used an emulsion process known as *collodain* process. **Frederick Scott Archer** (England,1951) is responsible for the discovery of wet collodion process. Wet collodion is a stichy substance, used as a binder for coating silver salts on glass. Emulsion plates were preferred in portrait photography. To have more focusing bellows were added to the cameras. The emulsion plates are classified as follows:
○ Ambrotype
○ Tintype

In ambro type, glass plate is used instead of copper plate. In tin type, tin plate is used. These plates are sensitive, compared to copper plates used in Daguerreotype. Many civil wars were photographed by using emulsion plates. To develop the plate, dark room with processing chemicals were needed. Hence, wagons were equipped and used with dark room facility. These plates were made according to the need, cannot be stored.

Dry Plates

In 1871, **Richard L. Maddox** (England) introduced dry gelatin silver bromide plates, instead of emulsion plates. The gelatin could dry on the plate without harming the silver salts. They are basically dry plates,

14 Medical X-ray Film Processing

offered equal quality and speed of emulsion plates. These plates can be made and stored for later use. Smaller camera with mechanical shutter was introduced. Hand-held camera came into the market with shorter of exposure time.

FLEXIBLE FILM

In 1880, **George Eastman** started a company **Kodak**. He invented a plate-coating machine; mostly on glass as well as paper (Fig. 1.5). Before that the plates were coated manually by hand. He used flexible roll films, instead of solid plates (1889). It is a transparent film made of cellulose nitrate to support the emulsion. This promoted the photography with availability of roll films. He made 100 exposures in a single roll film. His camera had a small lens, but there is no provision for focusing adjustment. The user should take the picture and return the camera to the factory for further development and printing. **Henri Cartier-Bresson** and others (1930) used 35 mm camera. It captured life images (as it occurs), instead of staggered photography. This was used extensively in the world war by the journalists to report the war images.

W. C. Roentgen had discovered X-rays on November 8, 1895. During that time, photography glass plates, flexible films and sensitized papers were available at the market. Roentgen realized the importance of photographic plate and had recorded his wife's hand (Fig. 1.6). Most of the radiographs were made by photographers or physicians interested in photography at that time. It was referred as *"new photography"* and several Roentgen's studios were established.

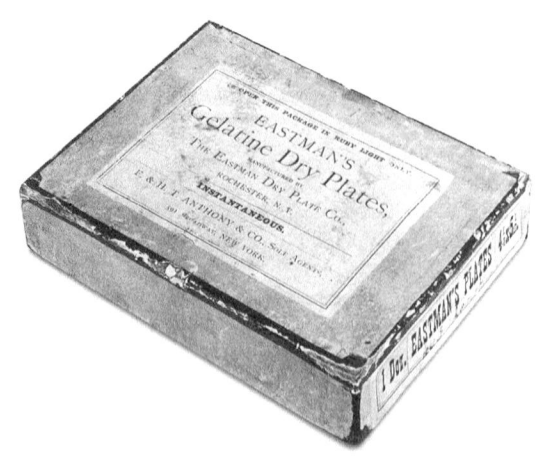

Fig. 1.5: Eastman's box containing gelatine dry plates.
(*Source*: Arthur G et al, Radiographics, 1989)

Fundamental Concepts 15

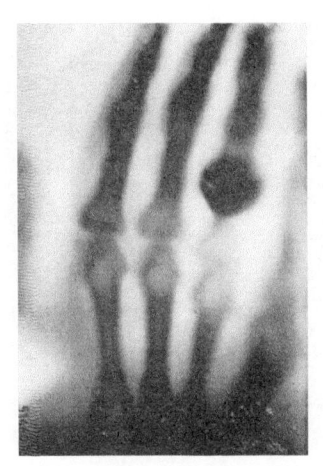

Fig. 1.6: First medical radiograph of Mrs. Roentgen's hand, made by WC Roentgen, 1895.
(*Source*: Arthur G et al. Radiographics, 1989)

After the Discovery of X-rays

Generally, it was thought that photography plates were superior than flexible films. However, the plates had the following limitations:
- No two were like
- The quantity of chemicals were not standardized
- Development was based on user's experience
- Low maximum density
- Lack of contrast
- Slow speed.

To address the above, photographic paper was introduced in 1886, especially for X-rays, but it failed without serving the purpose. **Dr.Carl Schienssner** (1896) made a German plate, by Roentgen's request. It had thicker emulsion and gave greater density for X-rays.

In 1896, **Thomas Edison** found that *calcium tungstate* is a fluorescent material and it is six times more intense than barium platinocyanide. He recommended calcium tungstate for X-ray work, especially for fluoroscopy examinations. **Prof. Michael Pupin** of Columbia University (1896) made the first radiograph with a fluorescent screen-film combination. He placed a fluorescent screen in contact with the photography plate and took a patient's hand (Fig. 1.7).

Meanwhile, the problems associated with fluorescent screens used with photography plates were realized as follows:
- Excessive graininess of large size crystal
- Non-uniformity of coating

16 Medical X-ray Film Processing

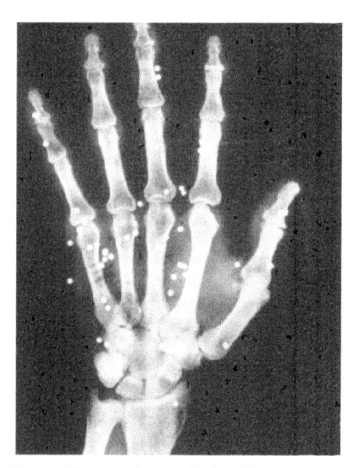

Fig. 1.7: First screen-film radiograph, made by Pupin, using intensifying screens.
(*Source*: Arthur G et al. Radiographics, 1989)

The photography plates were fragile, difficult for shipment, heavy (2 pounds) and expensive (1$). It can be coated at one side only. In addition, it has slow speed and lack in optimal density and contrast (Fig. 1.8). Since most of the plates were manufactured in **Belgium**, world war-I (1914), halted the production of photography plates. **Dr. Max Levy** (Germany) was the first, recommended the use of double–coated film between the intensifying screens (1897).

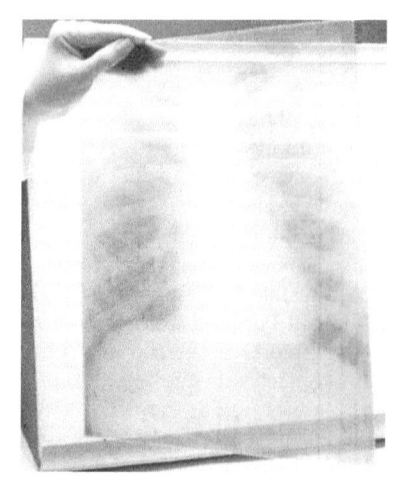

Fig. 1.8: First chest radiograph, recorded on a single-emulsion glass plate, 1912.
(*Source*: Arthur G et al. Radiographics, 1989)

In 1913, an X-ray film with cellulose nitrate base coated on one side was introduced. It was more sensitive to X-rays, required less exposure and is easy to use with intensifying screens. In 1916, a non-curling film base was introduced. **Carl V.S. Patterson** came with an improved intensifying screen, made up of calcium tungstate. It has minimal afterglow, improved uniformity and lesser impurity.

Screen-Film and Processor Developments

In 1918, double side emulsion film was introduced. This facilitated the use of two screens; front thin and back thick screens. However, there is some reluctance in the film processing, compared to plates. Since trays were used for processing and it is more convenient for plates than films. In 1920, film hangers and deep tanks (similar to present day manual processing tanks) were introduced for film processing.

In 1921, cleanable fluorescent screens were introduced with a thin protective coat at the top. This extended not only the life of screen, but also avoided the cost of replacement. In 1924, X-ray films with cellulose acetate base came in the market, which avoided the fire hazards of nitrate base film. In 1933, an X-ray film with a blue-tinted base was introduced. Subsequently, **Carl S.V. Patterson** (1934) developed *Par speed* screen. In 1936, non-screen X-ray film was introduced. It had higher speed, contrast and definition, compared to screen type films. It was common in 1930s, medical radiographs were taken by using pair of calcium tungstate intensifying screens with double emulsion X-ray films (Fig. 1.9).

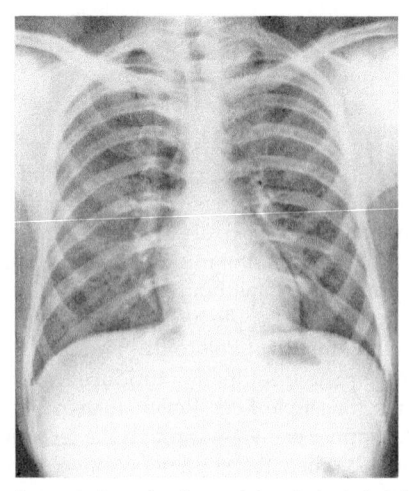

Fig. 1.9: Chest radiograph, by using two calcium tungstate intensifying screens with a double-emulsion medical X-ray film, 1945.
(*Source*: Arthur G et al. Radiographics, 1989)

Medical X-ray Film Processing

In 1948, barium lead sulfate phosphor screens were introduced. It provided greater speed than Par speed screens. X-ray film processing involves, developer, stop-bath, fixer, washing and drying. The user's processing time had controlled the final image quality, patient's exposure and reproducibility. To overcome this, the first prototype automatic X-ray film processor was introduced in 1942. Later (1956), first roller transport processor came, which completed the processing in 6 minutes. Automatic film processor has the following special features:
- Human error is avoided
- Helped to standardize techniques
- Lesser retakes
- Improved radiograph quality
- Patient waiting time reduced
- Efficiency and workflow improved.

In 1960, X-ray film with polyester base was introduced. Its advantage is that easy film handling, dimensional stability and improved film dry. In 1965, a 90 second automatic film processor came. In 1971, a newly designed screens and films with doubly curved paneled cassette were introduced. It improved screen-film contact, speed and definition. It used barium sulfate phosphor, which emits ultraviolet (UV) light for which the emulsion is more sensitive.

In 1972, a single side high resolution screen was introduced for mammography. This reduced the radiation exposure significantly. Rare-earth screens (1974) were introduced by **Finkel Stein** and **Wichersheim**. It had high absorption green emitting *gadolinium oxy-sulfide* phosphor. This is followed by *lanthanum oxy-bromide, yttrium oxy-sulfide* and *barium fluorochloride* phosphors. They become faster screens, due to their increased efficiency and absorption character.

Digital Photography

Polaroid came with a 35 mm camera (Model 95) and used a chemical process to develop film inside the camera. This was the birth of instant photography. Though it was very costly at the beginning, became cheaper at later period, due to the arrival of multiple models. However, Polaroid stopped the camera in 2008, without revealing the secret of instant photography. Though many people have tried to explore the secret, but none had achieved the quality of Polaroid.

The **Asahi**, the Japanese company introduced *Asahi flex SLR camera* in 1950. SLR stands for single Lens Reflex, it uses a mirror and prism system. The photographer can view through the lens and see the object, to be photographed. When the shutter button is pressed, the mirror flips out of the light path, permits the light to pass through the light receptor. At the same time, **Nikon** came with *Nikon F SLR camera*, with interchangeable lenses. These cameras were ruling the market over

40 years with multiple accessories and developments, including image control. In 1970, compact cameras came in the market. They are capable of making image control decision on their own. The camera calculates the shutter speed, aperture and focus, to take optimal photography. Hence, they are known as *automatic cameras* (point and shoot). SLR cameras are updated with the above facility.

There was a thinking to store images electronically (digital image) for long time. **Kodak** came with a digital camera in 1951, followed by **Canon, Nikon, Pentax** in the form of digital SLR (DSLR) cameras. Digital camera looks very much like ordinary film camera, but works differently from the film camera. The light path starting from the object, aperture and up to lens is the same in both cameras. In a film camera the emitted light from the object is incident on a light sensitive surface, inside the camera, which forms the latent image. The latent image is then developed into a visible image. The developed image is a negative one, because black area look like light and vice-versa. From the negative final image is printed, called as photo print. The photosensitive system is either a photographic plate or film.

The light detector used in the digital camera is either a *charge coupled device* (CCD) or *Complementary metal-oxide semiconductor* (CMOS) image sensor, which has a matrix size of 216 x 216--4064 x 2704. The smallest matrix element is called pixel, the detector is considered as divided into billions of pixels. In the case of megapixel camera one can have more than 20 million pixels. The image sensor is a micro chip with a width of 10 mm. The chip contains array of sensors, which convert the light into electrical signal. The emitted light of varying intensity from the object passes through the aperture and lens of the camera, is incident on the pixels and produce electrical charges. The sensor measures the electrical charge according to the color and brightness of each pixel and forms the electrical signal. This is converted into a digital data (binary number) and stored in a computer.

The first phone camera came in 2000 and nowadays smart phones are available with digital cameras. They offer very high quality photographic images.

2

Production of X-rays

DISCOVERY OF X-RAYS

X-rays were discovered by W.C. Roentgen, the German physicist in 1895, when he was investigating the conduction of electricity through gases at low pressure in glass tubes. He noticed that the positive electrodes in the tubes gave off invisible rays that caused fluorescent screens (barium platinocyanide screen kept near the tube) to glow and that fogged photographic plates. The rays were penetrating; they passed through black paper and even thicker objects. They were not deflected in electric and magnetic field. Therefore, Roentgen concluded that they were not charged particles. As their nature was not known he called them X-rays, later they were known to be electromagnetic radiation of very short wavelength. Roentgen received the first *Nobel Prize* in physics in 1901, for his discovery.

Properties of X-rays

- X-rays are electromagnetic radiations of shorter wavelength (0.1–10 nm).
- They travel in straight line with a velocity equal to light.
- X-rays are not influenced by electric and magnetic fields.
- X-rays penetrate through substances that are opaque to visible light.
- X-rays produce fluorescence in materials like *calcium tungstate* and *zinc-cadmium sulfide*.
- X-rays affect the photographic film and form latent image.
- X-rays produce ionization and excitation in the substances through which they pass.
- X-rays produce chemical changes in substances through which they pass.
- X-rays produce biological effects in living organisms. The cells can be either damaged or killed due to X-ray exposure.

Production of X-rays

X-rays are produced when fast moving electrons are stopped by means of a target material. The moving electron possesses kinetic energy. When the electron is suddenly stopped, its kinetic energy is converted into heat and X-rays. This conversion is taking place in the target material. Therefore, the interaction of electron with the target is the basis for X-ray production.

Electron Interaction with the Target

When the electron arrives at the target, it interacts in four ways as follows (Figs. 2.1A to D):
- Ionization of target atoms
- Characteristic X-rays
- Interaction with nuclear field
- Interaction with nucleus.

Ionization of target atoms: Fast moving electrons enter the surface layer of the target and undergo collisions. In this process, the incident electron transfers sufficient energy and removes an electron from the atom. This involves small energy transfer, resulting in ionization of target atoms. The incident electron may undergo number of such collisions and each time its direction gets altered. A 100 keV electron may encounter 1,000 of such interactions, before coming to rest and most of its energy appears as heat in the target. The displaced electron, known as a secondary electron, may have sufficient energy and produce further ionization of target atoms. They are few in number and produce their own track, known as *delta rays*.

Characteristic X-rays: This is an interaction between the incident electron and the electron in the K-shell. In this process, the incident electron directly hit the K-shell, transfers sufficient energy and removes the K-shell electron. The vacancy in the K-shell is filled by an electron moving inward from the outer shell. During this transition, the difference in binding energies of the two shells is given out as X-ray photon. This photon is known as the characteristic X-ray. The ejected electron may produce further interaction in other target atoms.

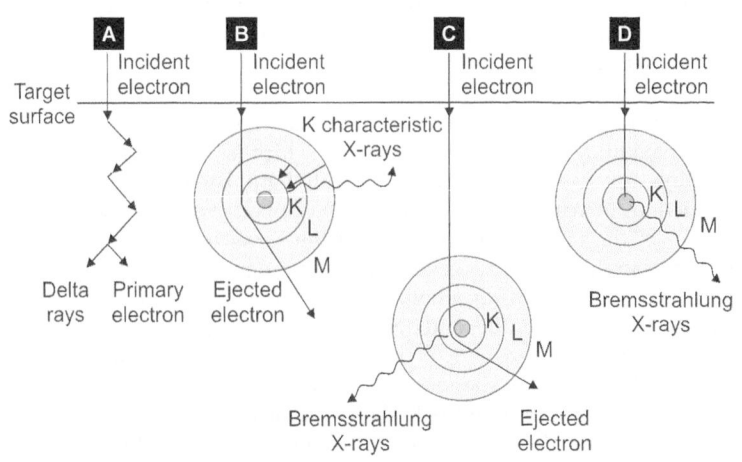

Figs. 2.1A to D: Interaction of electron with target atoms: (A) Ionization of target atoms; (B) Characteristic X-rays; (C) Interaction with nuclear field; and (D) Interaction with nucleus.

Interaction with nuclear field: The incident electron occasionally reaches nearer to the nucleus of an atom in the target. Since the electron is a negative particle, it is attracted by the positive nucleus. It is made to orbit partially around the nucleus, decelerates and goes out with reduced energy. The loss of energy appears in the form of X-ray photons, known as *bremsstrahlung*. In German, bremsstrahlung means breaking radiation. The maximum energy of the incident electron is determined by the applied voltage of the X-ray tube. An electron can lose all of its kinetic energy in the form of bremsstrahlung radiation. The energy of the X-ray photon depends on the degree to which the electron is decelerated by the nuclear attraction. The photon energy can take any value from zero to a maximum. This process is unlikely at low energies, but dominant at high energies.

Interaction with nucleus: The electron may hit the nucleus directly and is stopped completely in a single collision. The entire electron energy appears as bremsstrahlung radiation. This type of interaction is very rare, but capable of giving high energy X-rays.

In general, the interaction of B, C, and D are very rare in the diagnostic range of energies, leading to lesser amount of X-ray production (<1%). The ionizational collision (A) dominates (>99%) the interaction process and produces heat. Thus, the X-ray tube is inefficient in the conversion of electron energy into X-rays.

X-ray Spectra

X-ray photons produced by an X-ray tube are heterogeneous in energy. A graph drawn between the photon energy and X-ray intensity is called *X-ray spectrum*. There are two types of X-ray spectrum, namely:
○ Bremsstrahlung or continuous spectrum
○ Characteristic or line spectrum.

A bremsstrahlung spectrum consists of X-ray photons of all energies up to maximum in a continuous fashion, which is also known as white radiation, because of its similarity to white light. Bremsstrahlung X-ray production increases with increase of applied voltage and atomic number of the target material. Most of the X-ray imaging in hospitals are bremsstrahlung X-rays, except in mammography. A characteristic spectrum consists of X-ray photons of low energy. The position of the characteristic radiation depends upon the atomic number of the target. Only K-shell characteristic X-rays are very important in radiology. To eject a K-shell electron, the incident electron must have energy greater than the binding energy of the K-shell. Characteristic X-rays occur only at discrete energy levels, capable of producing *Auger electrons*. It finds application mammography imaging.

The intensity of the X-rays can be plotted against photon energy in a graph (Fig. 2.2). The area under the curve is proportional to the total

Production of X-rays

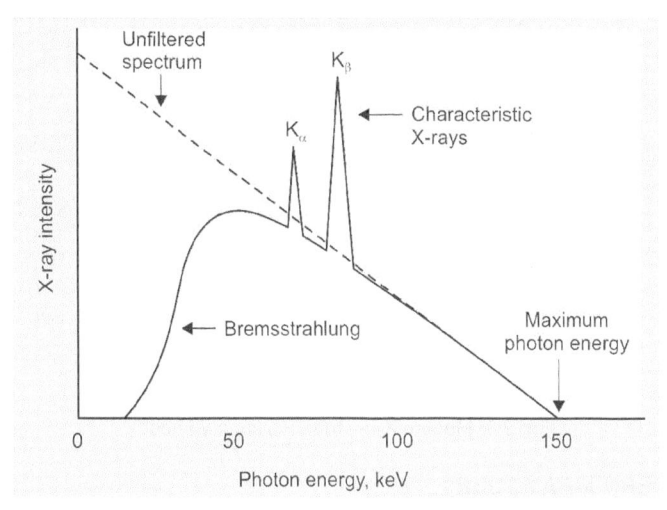

Fig. 2.2: X-ray spectrum consisting bremsstrahlung and characteristic X-rays.

number of photons emitted. The highest X-ray energy is determined by the peak voltage (kV$_p$) applied in the X-ray tube. The characteristic spectrum is superimposed on the continuous spectrum. An unfiltered beam spectrum (theoretical) will be a straight line and mathematically given by **Kramer's** equation:

$$I_E = KZ(E_m - E)$$

where, I_E is the intensity of photons with energy E, Z is the atomic number of the target, E_M is the maximum photon energy and K is a constant. The unfiltered X-ray spectrum looks like a ramp.

In practice, the X-ray beam is a filtered beam, due to inherent and added filtration. The filtration hardens the beam, by absorbing the low energy X-rays up to 10 keV, which is evident by the bremsstrahlung spectrum in the graph. The number of photons increase initially, with photon energy and later decrease linearly up to maximal photon energy. The X-ray spectrum is influenced by the following factors:

- Applied voltage
- Target material
- Tube current
- Exposure time
- Bremsstrahlung process
- Filtration.

To specify the quality of X-rays, a rule of thumb is used, which states that the effective energy is about 1/3 to 1/2 of maximum X-ray energy. K-shell characteristic X-ray contribution is about 10% at 100 kV photon energy. There is no presence of characteristic X-ray at <70 kV.

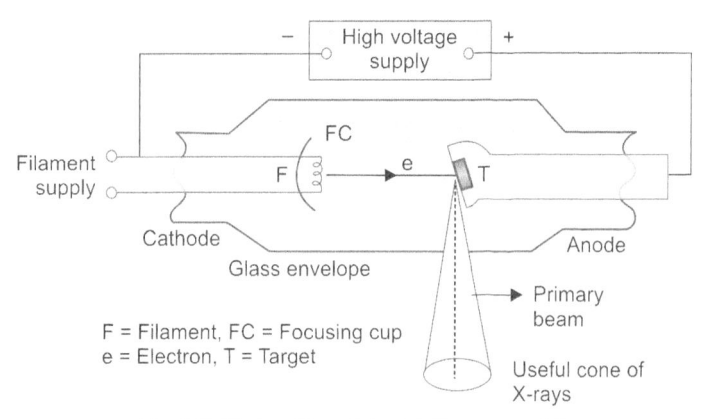

Fig. 2.3: Modern X-ray tube (stationary anode).

MODERN X-RAY TUBE

In earlier periods gas tubes were used to produce X-rays. But these tubes suffered with disadvantages. Hence, **Coolidge** proposed a prototype X-ray tube based on the thermionic emission principle (1913). On the basis of Coolidge tube, several X-ray tubes have been designed. The stationary anode X-ray tube is one of the modern X-ray tube in which the anode is stationary.

The stationary anode X-ray tube consists a cathode and an anode, which are kept in an evacuated glass bulb made up of Pyrex glass (Fig. 2.3). This is kept in a housing that provides insulation, cooling (oil) and shielding to leakage radiation. The primary X-ray emerges through the window. The cathode consists of a tungsten filament in the form of a coil placed in a shallow focusing cup. The filament is made of tungsten wire, about 0.2 mm in diameter, that is coiled to form a vertical spiral about 0.2 cm in diameter and 1 cm in length. The filament is heated by passing an electric current (10 V,4A) through it from a low voltage supply. Sometimes, one can have two filaments in a single tube, to have two focal spots.

The anode is made of copper block in which a small tungsten plate is embedded. The tungsten is a square or rectangular plate of 2 mm or 3 mm thick and the dimension is greater than 1 cm. The tungsten plate serves as a target. The target is positioned at online focus principle, in order to increase the ratio of the actual focal area to the effective focal area. The area of the target in which the electron bombards and produce X-rays is called *focal spot*. It is viewed by the patient direction. There may be small and large focal area. Small focal spot produces sharp images with good spatial resolution. Large focal spot is recommended for high heat loading and short exposures. Typical focal spot size range is about 0.1 to 1.2 mm.

The anode angle is usually 7–20°. A high voltage supply is applied between the cathode and anode to accelerate the electrons. A vacuum of the order of 10^{-5} mm Hg is maintained in the tube.

When the filament is heated to white light, it emits electrons by thermionic emission principle. The focusing cup (made up of nickel) produces an electric field that focuses the electron to the focal area. The focusing cup also protects the adjacent parts of the tube wall from damage by electron bombardment. If the anode is made positive with respect to the filament, these electrons will be attracted to the anode. This will constitute an electron current around the circuit in the anticlockwise direction. The tube current is measured by the milliammeter (mA). Usually, there is an electron cloud (space charge) between the anode and cathode. The applied voltage should overcome the electron cloud, then only current flows in the tube. The minimum applied potential to create the tube current is 40 kV. Tube current increases with filament heating/current. The tube current ranges from 1–1200 mA.

Since the space between anode and cathode is a high vacuum, the electrons do not collide with gas molecules in crossing the gap and so acquire very high velocities. The electrons which are accelerated by the applied voltage possess high kinetic energy. When they suddenly stopped in the target, X-rays are emitted in all directions. About one-half of these are absorbed in the target itself. The remaining portion emerges as a useful primary X-ray beam. During the production of X-rays, large amount of heat is produced in the target. The tube is also provided with suitable cooling system to remove the heat very quickly.

Stationary anode tubes have a small target area that limits the heat dissipation and this limits the X-ray output. Dental X-ray units, portable X-ray units, and portable fluoroscopy systems use stationary anode X-ray tubes. Alternatively, rotating anode X-ray tubes are used in mammography, cardiac catheterization laboratory and CT scans. These tubes employ rotor and induction motor to rotate the anode, thereby increasing the effective target area and heat capacity.

Quality and Intensity of X-rays

Quality

The term quality describes the penetrating power of the radiation. If a radiation consists of photons of single energy (monoenergetic), then the quality can be described either by photon energy or wavelength. But X-ray beam consists of many photon energies (heterogeneous), and hence, its quality cannot be described by the photon energy. Therefore, the X-ray beam quality is usually specified by the following:
- Half-value layer (HVL)
- Applied voltage (kV)
- Filtration
- Effective photon energy.

Medical X-ray Film Processing

Half-value Layer

The half value layer (HVL) or half-value thickness (HVT) of a radiation beam is the required thickness of a material which reduces the beam intensity to one half. The HVL is always stated together with the value of the applied voltage and the filtration. *Aluminum* and *copper* are the materials commonly used to specify HVL.

Intensity

The intensity is a measure of quantity of radiation, that is the number of X-rays in the beam. The intensity of a radiation beam is the energy flowing in unit time through a unit area. It is equal to the number of photons in the beam multiplied by the energy of each photon. The intensity is commonly measured in roentgens per minute (R min^{-1}) or air kerma (mGy). The X-ray intensity is proportional to the tube current (Fig. 2.4A) and exposure time. Doubling the tube current or exposure time will double the X-ray beam intensity. The product of tube current (mA) and exposure time (s), is called mAs. The mAs affects the beam intensity, not the photon energy.

Increase of kV also increases X-ray beam intensity in a quadratic manner (Fig. 2.4B). It also increases the photon energy. Any variation in the applied voltage will change the shape of the X-ray spectrum. The maximum photon energy is determined by the applied voltage.

The term exposure is often used in radiology, which is proportional to the energy fluence of the X-ray beam. It refers both quality and quantity of the beam. The term quantity refers the number of X-ray photons in the beam.

Filter

A filter is a metallic sheet introduced in the path of X-rays, in order to reduce the patient dose. Diagnostic X-rays consist of both low energy and high energy. When X-rays pass through a patient, only high energy X-rays penetrate through the patient and form the radiological image. However, the low energy X-rays are absorbed in the first few cm of tissue, thereby increasing the radiation dose. The introduction of filters absorb these low energy X-rays and reduce the patient dose. This process of removing the low energy X-rays, by introducing metallic sheets is called *filtration* (Fig. 2.5). Filtration has two components namely:
- Inherent filtration
- Added filtration.

Filtration resulting from the absorption of X-rays by the X-ray tube and its housing is called inherent filtration. It usually varies between 0.5 to 1.0 mm of Al equivalent. Added filtration results from absorbers placed externally in the path of the X-ray beam. The sum of the inherent and added filtration gives the total filtration:

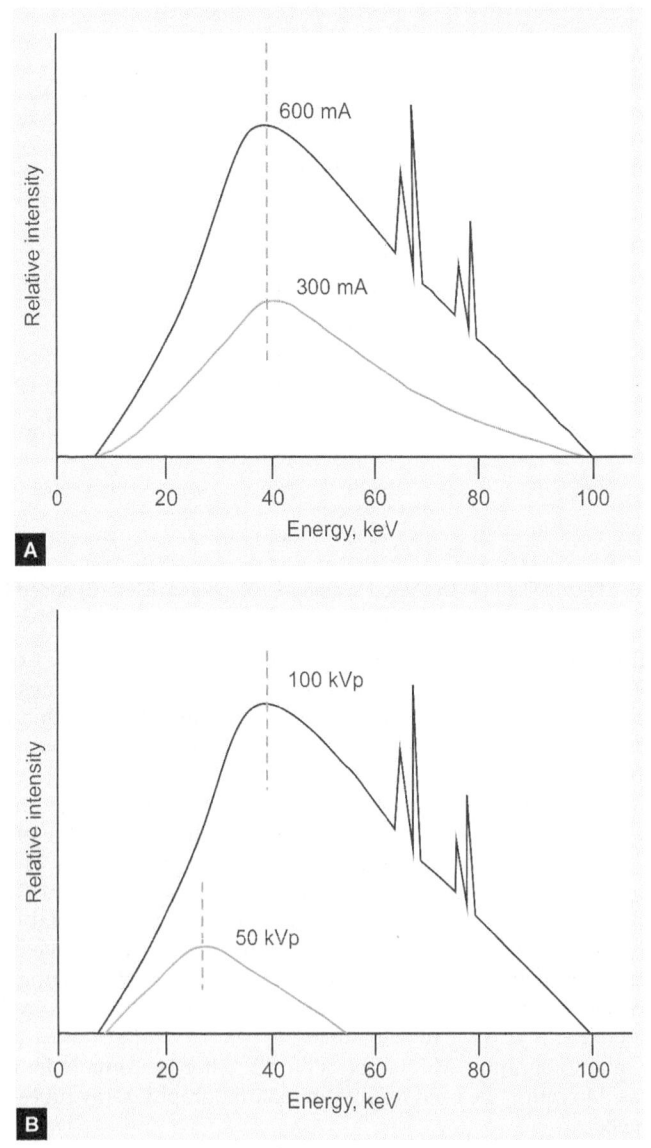

Figs. 2.4A and B: Effect of: (A) tube current (mA); (B) applied voltage (kV).

Total filtration = Inherent filtration + Added filtration.

Al and Cu are the materials usually used in diagnostic radiology. The thickness of added filter varies from 1.0 to 1.5 mm of Al. Aluminum

28 Medical X-ray Film Processing

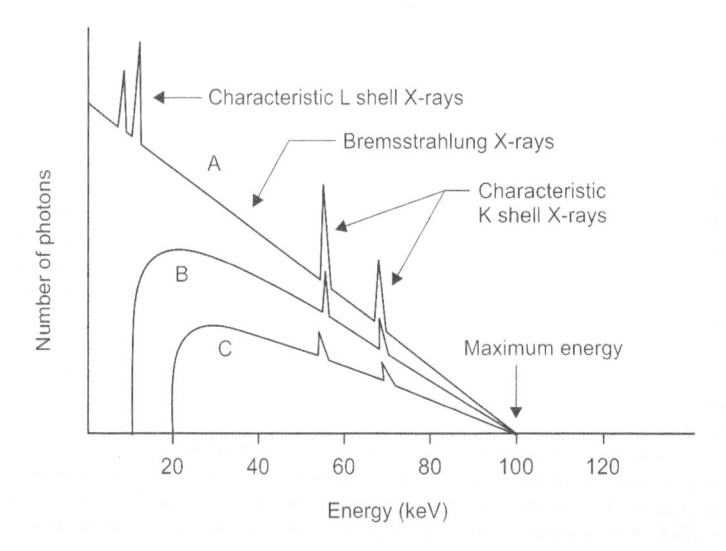

Fig. 2.5: Effect of filter: (A) Unfiltered spectrum; (B) inherent filter; (C) added filter.

(Z = 13) is an excellent filter material for low energy X-rays. Copper (Z = 29) is a better filter for high energy radiation. Copper is always used in combination with aluminum as a compound filter. A compound filter consists of two or more layers of different metals. The layers are arranged in such a way that the high Z layer always faces the X-ray tube.

The recommended total filtration for diagnostic X-ray unit of >70 kVp is 2.5 mm Al. X-ray units with proper filter, reduces the patient dose significantly, up to 80%. Filters are simple and inexpensive. Though filters reduce the intensity of X-ray beam significantly, it does not affect the maximum energy of the X-ray beam spectrum. Heavy metal filters (Gd, Ho) are also used in general radiography. These filters make use of the K-edge, and offer increased absorption of X-rays, while imaging with contrast agents. They enhance contrast for iodine and barium, reduce patient dose and increase tube loading.

In mammography Mo target with Rh filter is commonly used, whereas, Mo cannot be used as filter in mammography X-ray tubes with Rh targets.

Beam Restrictor/Collimator

An X-ray beam restrictor is a device that is attached to the X-ray tube housing, to regulate the size and shape of an X-ray beam. They can be classified into three categories namely:

Production of X-rays

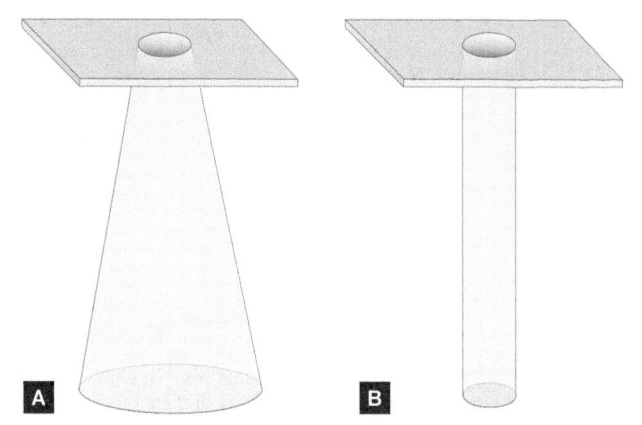

Figs. 2.6A and B: Beam restrictors: (A) Cone; (B) Cylinder.

- Aperture diaphragm
- Cone and cylinder
- Collimator.

Aperture diaphragm consists of a sheet of lead with a hole in the center. The size of the hole determines the size and shape of the X-ray beam. It is simple and the aperture can be altered to any size and shape. The disadvantage of an aperture diaphragm is that it produces large penumbra. The penumbra can be reduced by keeping the aperture diaphragm far away from the X-ray target. Aperture diaphragm is used in dental radiography with rectangular collimation. In addition, it is used in trauma and chest radiography.

The use of cone and cylinder will reduce the penumbra considerably (Figs. 2.6A and B). Both have extended metal structures that restrict the useful circular beam to the required size. The position and size of the distal end determine the field size. If the X-ray source, cone and film are not aligned properly, then one side of the film may not be exposed, which is called as *cone cutting*. Cone is a ideal beam restrictor, but the flare of the cone is greater than the flare of the X-ray beam. These systems provide only limited number of field sizes.

The collimator is the best X-ray beam restrictor. It defines the size and shape of the X-ray field that emerges from the X-ray tube. The collimator assembly is attached to the tube housing at the tube port. A collimator consists of two sets of shutters, which can be moved independently. Each shutter consists of four or more lead plates, which can absorb X-rays completely, to provide a well defined X-ray field. When the shutters are closed, they meet at the center of the X-ray field.

The collimator also has a light and mirror arrangement, to illuminate the X-ray field. The light bulb is positioned laterally and the mirror is

30 Medical X-ray Film Processing

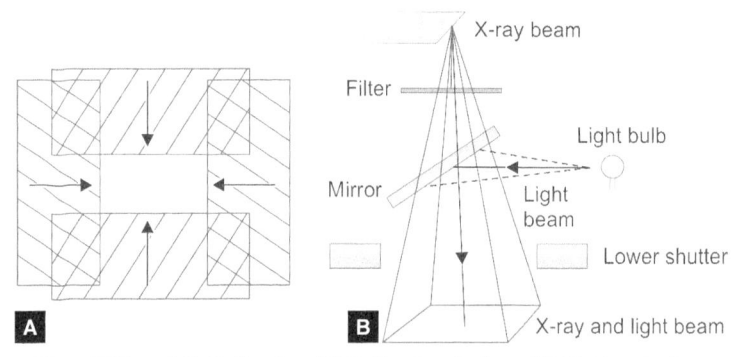

Figs. 2.7A and B: Collimator: (A) Collimator shutters; (B) Light and mirror arrangement for the alignment of X-ray and light field.

mounted in the path of the X-ray beam at an angle 45° (Figs. 2.7A and B). The target and the light bulb should be kept at equal distance from the center of the mirror. The collimator provides variety of rectangular X-ray fields and the light beam shows the center of the X-ray field. The light field and radiation field should match exactly with each other. The variation must be within 4% of target to film distance (TFD). The alignment of light beam and X-ray beam should be checked periodically. A well collimated beam, cover lesser area of the patient, giving less patient dose. It also generates less scatter radiation, which improves the image quality.

Collimator that automatically limits the X-ray field size to the useful area of the detector is also available. These are called *positive beam limitation (PBL)* collimators. A sensor in the cassette holder, adjust the collimator opening, equal to the cassette dimensions. Thus, PBL collimator limits the irradiated volume and reduces the patient dose.

Scattered Radiation and Grid

When the beam of X-rays pass through the patient, the beam is absorbed and scattered. The absorbed primary beam gives a useful shadow, while the scattered radiation will tend to spoil the shadow. Scattered radiation contributes a constant background fog to the film image. This will increase the noise in the image. The ratio between the amounts of scattered radiation energy to the amount of primary radiation energy at a point is called scatter to primary ratio (SPR). The SPR increases with thicker patient and larger field size. For example, in abdomen radiography, only 20% of the photons contributes to the image formation and the other 80% goes as scattered radiation. Hence, scattered radiation must be removed, in order to increase the image contrast.

The scattered radiation can be removed by a grid, placed in-between the film and the patient. The grid consists of a series of parallel lead or tantalum strips of thickness **c** (50 µm) and of height **h** separated by spacers

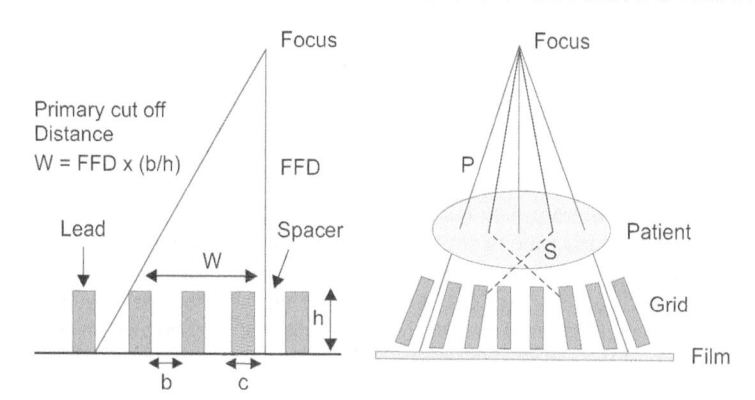

Fig. 2.8: Grid design and principle.

of low attenuating material of width **b** (350 μm) as shown in Figure 2.8. Aluminum or plastic fibers are used as low attenuating spacers. The grid is positioned between the patient and the detector, so that its long axis is pointed towards the X-ray beam. The primary X-rays coming out of the patient, passes through the inter space, since it is parallel in direction. The scattered X-rays, which are in non-parallel direction, strike the grid bars and being absorbed. The ratio of the primary transmission to the scatter transmission of a grid is called the *selectivity*.

Grid Ratio

The ability of the grid to discriminate against scattered radiation is measured by the grid ratio, which is defined as the ratio of the height to the width of the spacer between the lead strips.

$$\text{Grid ratio} = h/b$$

As the grid ratio increases, the grid removes more scatter radiations. The strip line density is $1/(b+C)$ lines per unit length. Typical grid ratio ranges from 4:1 to 16:1 and strip line densities from 25 to 60 lines per cm. The performance of a grid can be understood by *contrast improvement factor*. It is the ratio between image contrast with grid and image contrast without grid at 100 kVp. Higher grid ratio provides higher contrast improvement factor. However, it increases patient dose, as it employs higher exposure techniques. *Bucky factor* (**Gustave Bucky, 1913**) is another parameter which relates to the patient dose. It is the ratio between the patient dose with grid and patient dose without grid. Bucky factor increases with increase of kVp and grid ratio.

Types of Grid

Grids may be classified as:
- Parallel grid
- Crossed grid

- Focused grid
- Moving grid (Potter-Bucky).

In a parallel grid the lead strips are parallel to each other in their longitudinal axis. Most of the X-ray tables are provided with parallel grids. It is easy to design, but has the property of *grid cut off*. This means that the attenuation of primary radiation is greater at the edges and it can be partial or complete cut off. The distance of grid cut off may be estimated from the ratio of source to image distance (SID) to grid ratio.

Crossed grid is made up of lead strips that are parallel to the long axis and short axis of the grid. Usually, it is designed with two parallel grids, that are perpendicular each other. The grid ratio of crossed grids is equal to the sum of the ratios of the two parallel grids. Crossed grid is efficient in removing scatter radiations and has higher contrast improvement factor, and high grid ratio. It is useful at high kVp and tilt-table exposure techniques. The disadvantages include, difficulty in positioning, proper alignment of tube and table, and higher patient dose. Crossed grid also suffers from grid cut off. Focused grid is made mainly to reduce grid cut off. The lead strip lies in a imaginary radial lines of a circle, whose centre is the focal spot. The strips are parallel to the divergence of the X-ray beam. The grids are marked with focal distance and the side facing the target. If it is reversed, grid cut off may occur, hence, enough care is needed to position focused grid.

Moving Grid

When a focused or parallel grid is used, each lead strip will appear on the radiograph as very fine line. These lines may spoil the information in the film. However, these lines may be removed by moving the grid during the radiographic exposure. This is the principle of Potter-Bucky grid (**Hollis E. Potter**, 1920). Generally, focused grids are used as moving grids. The grid is made to move continuously in one direction. The grid motion is timed by the exposure control of the X-ray machine. It starts moving just before the X-rays are turned ON and continues to move even after the exposure is OFF. The traveling period of the grid should be greater than the exposure time. There are two types of moving grids namely:
- Reciprocating grid
- Oscillating grid.

The reciprocating is driven by a motor and the grid moves back and forth several times, during exposure. The distance traveled may be of the order of 2 cm. In the oscillating type, the grid is kept in a frame, which has 2–3 cm clearance on all sides. An electromagnet pulls and releases the grid before the exposure. The grid oscillates in circular path about the frame and comes to rest after 20–30 seconds.

Moving grids increases the distance between patient and film, resulting magnification, cassette motion and image blur. However, the

Production of X-rays

motion blur is undetectable, therefore used widely. The use of grid will always increase the exposure, because it will absorb some of the primary radiation. Therefore, in order to reduce the exposures, grids with smaller ratios are preferred. Generally, low ratio grids such as 8:1, is used with energies up to 90 kVp. High ratio grids such as 12:1 are preferred for high energy radiation. These grids produce films with better contrast with increased patient dose. Grids are generally used for body parts >12 cm thick or techniques >70 kVp. Grid can produce artifacts when improperly aligned.

Air Gap Techniques

Air gap technique is an alternative method of eliminating scatter radiation with large radiographic fields. When X-ray beam passes through the patient, it gets scattered in all directions. The intensity of scatter radiation is maximum at the patient's surface and decreases rapidly at increasing distance from the surface. If sufficient gap is allowed between the patient and film, this scattered photon will not reach the film. Higher focus to film distance (FFD) is used with air gap techniques, in order to maintain image sharpness. Hence, it requires greater exposure factors compared to grid. However, the patient exposures are generally low, due to higher FFD. Air gaps technique also introduce magnification. Air gap technique is most effective, when the point of scatter exists closer to the film. Air gaps techniques are used for Neuro-radiography and mammography.

INTERACTION OF RADIATION WITH MATTER

Attenuation

When radiation passes through a medium, it is partly absorbed, scattered and partly transmitted through the medium. The term attenuation refers both absorption and scattering. The attenuation is due to interaction of radiation with the medium. As a result, the intensity of radiation decreases exponentially. This means that the first few centimeters of the medium attenuate the radiation heavily, whereas later thickness attenuates relatively lesser. To attenuate the radiation completely, one must have infinite thickness of the medium. Hence, the intensity of transmitted radiation is always lesser than the incident radiation. If a photon passes through an absorber of thickness X (Figs. 2.9A and B), then the incident and transmitted radiation intensity is related as follows:

$$I = I_0 \, e^{-\mu x} \text{ or } \mu x = \log(I_0/I)$$

where, I is the transmitted photon intensity, I_0 is the incident photon intensity, e is the base of natural logarithm and μ is the linear attenuation coefficient of the medium. The negative sign indicates the reduction of radiation intensity.

Medical X-ray Film Processing

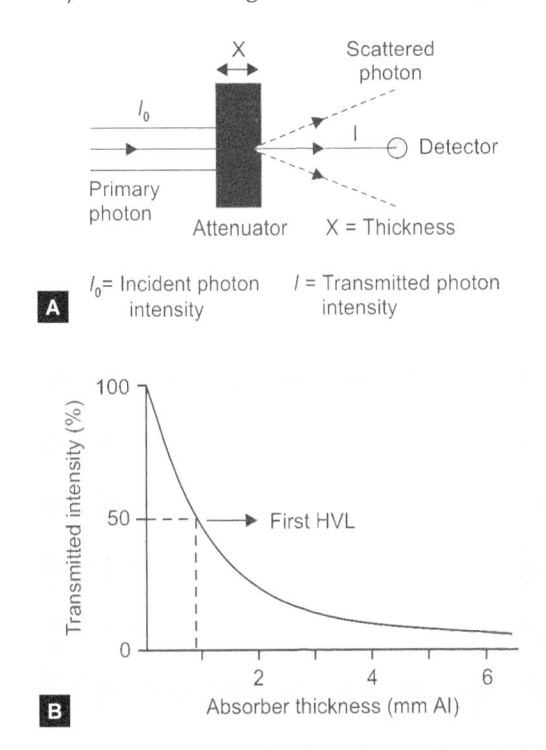

Figs. 2.9A and B: (A) Attenuation of radiation in a medium of thickness X; (B) Graph shows that the attenuation is exponential in nature. (HVL: Half-value layer)

Linear Attenuation Coefficient

The linear attenuation coefficient (μ) is defined as the reduction of radiation intensity per unit path length and it is expressed in cm^{-1}. This means that the μ is the amount of photons removed in one centimeter travel in the medium. It depends on the medium density and energy of the radiation. Different radiation energy is attenuated differently by a same medium. Same radiation can be attenuated differently by different medium. The linear attenuation coefficient concept is very much useful to understand CT scan principle and room shielding design in radiation safety.

Mass Attenuation Coefficient

Mass attenuation coefficient (μ/ρ) is the ratio of linear attenuation coefficient and density. It is obtained by dividing the linear attenuation coefficient by the density of the medium. The advantage is that, it becomes density-independent and its unit is square meter per kilogram ($m^2 kg^{-1}$).

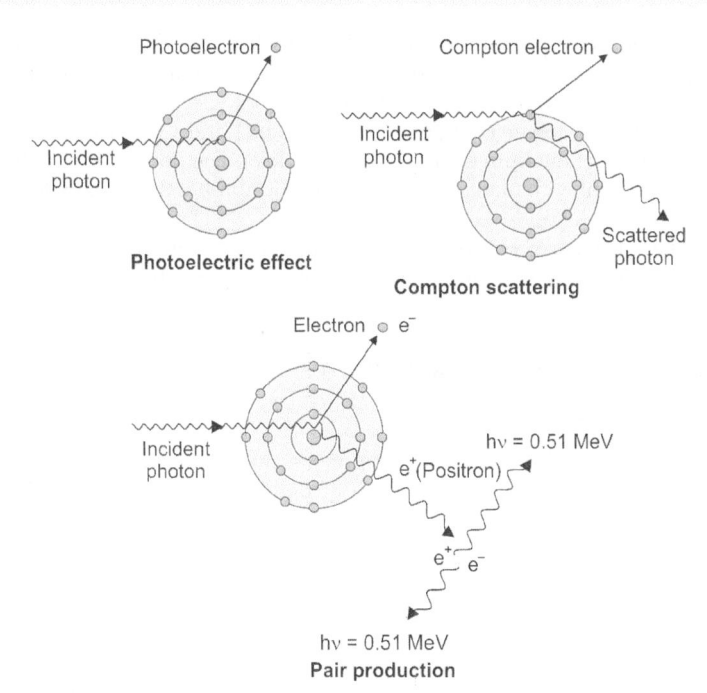

Fig. 2.10: Interactions of radiation with matter.

Interactions with Matter

The predominant modes of interaction of X-rays and gamma rays with mediums are *photoelectric effect* and *Compton effect* (Fig. 2.10). In photoelectric effect, the photon interacts with a bound electron (innermost orbit electron) of the medium and transfers its entire energy to the electron. The orbital electron is knocked out. This is known as *photoelectron* which will be absorbed in the medium itself. The probability of this interaction:
- Decreases with increase in energy of the incident radiation
- Increases with increase in atomic number of the medium.

This means that in a medium, the probability of photoelectric effect is more for 0.1 MeV photon, compared to that of 1 MeV photon. The photons undergo photoelectric effect, more readily in lead than in iron.

In Compton effect, the photon interacts with free electron (electron in the outermost orbit), and transfers a part of its energy to the electron. The photon, after interaction, travels in a different direction and will be called *scattered photon*. The probability of this interaction:
- Decreases with increase in energy of the incident photon
- Does not vary much with atomic number of the medium.

Although the probabilities of both photoelectric and Compton effect decrease with increase in photon energy, the decrease is more steep in the case of photoelectric effect. Hence, photoelectric effect is more predominant at lower energies (up to 500 keV) and Compton effect is predominant at medium energies (up to 5 MeV). The photoelectric effect is predominant with material of higher atomic number than that of lower atomic number.

The intensity of photons reduces on passing through any material. This is known as attenuation, which follows an exponential law, as stated above.

RADIATION QUANTITIES AND UNITS

Becquerel/Curie

Radioactivity is measured in terms of the number of transformations taking place in one second. The unit of radioactivity is Becquerel (Bq), corresponding to one transformation per second. The earlier unit of radioactivity was *curie* (Ci), equal to 3.7×10^{10} transformations per second.

Roentgen

The term exposure is used to obtain information about quantity of X or gamma radiations present at a point of interest, based on the ability of radiation to produce ionization in air. The unit of exposure is coulomb per kilogram (C/kg). The old unit of exposure was roentgen (R), which is equal to 2.58×10^{-4} C/kg.

Gray/Rad

Dose is the energy imparted by ionizing radiations in unit mass of the exposed material. The unit of dose is joule per kilogram (J/kg), which is called as gray (Gy). The old unit of dose was rad, stands for Radiation Absorbed Dose. One rad corresponds to an energy absorption of 100 ergs per gram in the exposed material. One gray is equal to 100 rads.

Kerma

Kerma stands for "kinetic energy released in the medium", which describes the initial interaction of the photon with an atom in the medium. When X-and gamma rays pass through a medium, they transfer kinetic energy to the charged particles (electrons and protons). Kerma (K) is the measure of kinetic energy transferred to the charged particles, at the initial phase. The unit for Kerma is also joule per kilogram (J kg^{-1}). The System International (SI) unit is gray and the special unit is rad. When the reference material is air, the quantity is called *"air kerma"*.

Sievert/Rem

The biological damage to tissue depends on the type of radiation. With the same dose, alpha radiation can cause 20 times more damage as gamma radiations. Hence, radiation requires a weight-age, to account its biological effects damage. The quantity equivalent dose takes into account the biological damage caused by the type of radiations. The product of the absorbed dose and radiation weighting factor is called *equivalent dose (H)*:

$$H = D \times W_R$$

where, D is the absorbed dose and W_R is the weighting factor for the radiation type (Table 2.1). The weighting factor is 1 for X-rays, gamma rays, and electron of all energies. High linear energy transfer (LET) radiation may cause higher biological effect, hence, have higher radiation weighting factor. The SI unit of equivalent dose is sievert (Sv) and 1 Sv = 1 J/kg. *Rem* is the special unit of equivalent dose, used early, when absorbed dose is measured in rad. Rem is the short form of radiation equivalent men and 100 rem is equal 1 Sv.

To account for the variation of radiosensitivity of different tissues and the nonuniformity of radiation exposure, International Commission on Radiological Protection (ICRP) has established tissue weighting factors (W_T). The weighting factor of a particular tissue or organ (Table 10.2, Chapter 10) has the risk of stochastic effects being induced in the organ when singly irradiated, compared to the total risk of inducing stochastic effects, if the same radiation dose is received by the whole body. The sum of the products of the equivalent dose to each tissue irradiated (H_T) and the corresponding weighting factor of tissue is called the *effective dose (E)*:

$$E = \Sigma\, W_T \times H_T$$

where, W_T is the weighting factor of tissue T and H_T is the mean equivalent dose received by the tissue T.

In addition, there are two more quantities, which are very important in diagnostic X-rays. They are potential difference (kV) and milliampere (mA). The potential difference applied between the cathode and the anode in

Table 2.1: Radiation weighting factors (W_R), (ICRP-103, 2007).

Radiation type	W_R
Photons (X and γ rays)	1
Electrons and muons	1
Protons and pions	2
Alpha particles, fission fragments, heavy ions	20
Neutrons	Continuous curve as a function of neutron energy

an X-ray machine is expressed in terms of kilovoltage. When the 200 kV potential difference is applied, the energy of X-rays produced varies from 0 kev to 200 keV. Higher the applied kV, higher is the energy of X-rays emitted and higher is the penetration power of X-rays. With increase in kV, the intensity of X-ray also increases. The milliampere of an X-ray unit indicates the current flowing through the tube. The intensity of X-rays increases with increase in mA. Thus, both kV and mA influence intensity, whereas kV only influences quality of X-rays.

X-RAY IMAGES

X-rays can readily penetrate through matter, and it depends upon X-ray energy, material density and atomic number. When X-ray passes through human body, bones absorb more X-rays than soft tissue and air cavity. As a result, the transmitting radiation is less under bone, more under soft tissue, and highest under air cavity. This transmitted intensity distribution of X-rays is recorded in a film. This X-ray film gives the image, which is known as *radiograph*. The final image is a two-dimensional picture made up of variety of black, white and gray superimposed shadows. Bones appear white and soft tissue appears as black in the radiograph. The white or radiopaque shadows on a film represent dense object, which offer total attenuation to X-rays. The black or radiolucent shadows represent object which has transmitted all the X-rays. The gray shadows represent areas where the X-ray beams have been stopped to a varying degree (Fig. 2.11).

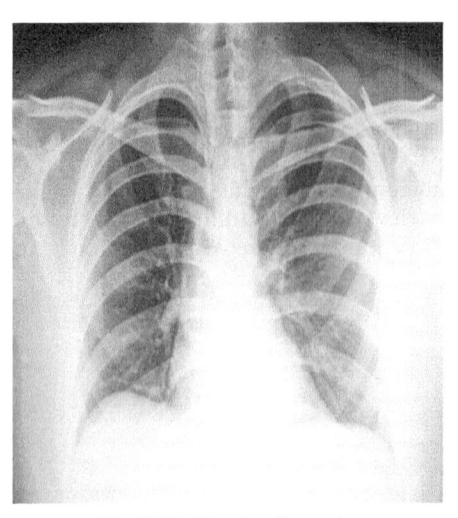

Fig. 2.11: Chest radiograph.

3
Medical X-ray Film

FILM STRUCTURE

The transmitted X-rays from the patient should be converted into visible image to the human eye for interpretation. The device that does the job is called *image receptor*. The image receptors are *X-ray film, fluorescent screen* and *solid state devices*. The medical X-ray film is used for capturing, displaying and storing radiographic images. It consists of the following parts:
- Base
- Adhesive layer
- Emulsion
- Overcoat

The emulsion is coated on both sides and hence, it is called double side emulsion film (Fig. 3.1).

Base

The base gives a rigid support on which the emulsion is coated. It should also be sufficiently transparent for viewing the radiograph clearly.

It should be flexible, fracture-resistant, and easy to handling without kinking. The base used should be dimensionally stable to maintain uniform image stability during processing and storage. It should be sufficiently firm and rigid to avoid kinking. It should have uniform lucency and transparent to light. It should be inert, so that the sensitometric properties of the emulsion are not affected.

Initially, glass and *cellulose nitrate* were used as bases. Later, the base *cellulose triacetate* (CTA) and *polyester* are being introduced. CTA is the safety base introduced by **George Eastman** in 1920 for the first time. Polyester (1960) is made from polyethylene terephthalate resin. Polyester

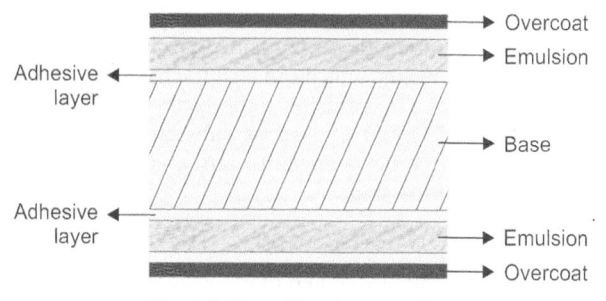

Fig. 3.1: X-ray film cross-section.

base is resistant to warping from age, stronger with higher dimensional stability. It is thinner in size (175 μm) and easy to transport in automatic film processor. The polyester base has many advantages as follows:
- Dimensional stability
- Optical clarity
- Waterproof
- High tensile strength
- Flexible
- Chemical memory
- Inert to processing chemicals.

The base is generally 180 microns thick in the case of CTA and 160 microns thick in the case of polyester. The thickness should be uniform, otherwise variations in the depth of emulsion layer may occur. The base should be free from all blemishes. The base can either be colored or clear. Blue-based films give the following benefits:
- It gives pleasing image
- It is much more restful on the viewer's eye in continuous viewing
- It also gives higher visual contrast.

The main disadvantage is presence of high-base fog, when the film is viewed on a poor quality view box (yellow light emission).

Clear base has a very low-base fog and lower visual contrast. Continued viewing may be more tiresome for some viewers. Because of lower base fog, this film is suitable for ultrasound work.

The X-ray film base is usually added with a dye, so that the film looks like blue. These films are called blue tinted, which reduces eye strain and fatigue. It gives pleasing appearance to the intermediate densities in the image and increases the diagnostic accuracy. Both CTA and polyester come under the class of safety bases. Both have sufficient dimensional stability for all radiographic purposes, although polyester has a higher tear resistance.

Adhesive Layer

The adhesive layer (*substratum*) lies in between the base and emulsion, in the form of thin coat. It uniformly binds the emulsion layer to the base. The choice of material depends on the nature of the base material. The substratum contains solvents, which can etch the base and thus provides sufficient anchorage for the emulsion to be coated on it subsequently. Usually, monolayer of *gelatin* is used as substratum. It also helps to maintain proper contact between emulsion and base, and provide integrity during film processing.

Emulsion

The emulsion (3–5 μm thick) is coated over the adhesive layer. Emulsion consists of gelatin medium and light sensitive silver halide crystal in a

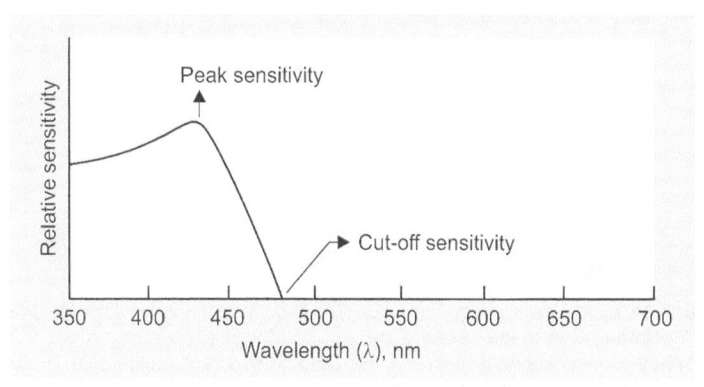

Fig. 3.2: Spectrogram of silver bromide (AgBr).

uniform manner. Gelatin is transparent to light and porous for chemicals. It gives support for silver halide, by holding them properly. Among the halides, *silver bromide* (98%) and *silver iodide* (2%) is used as crystal in the film. These halides are flat and have high atomic numbers; bromide (Z = 35), silver (Z = 47), and iodide (Z = 53), compared to gelatin (Z = 7). The halide crystals are available in *tabular, cubic, octahedral, polyhedral,* or irregular grain shapes. Tabular grain shape (thickness 0.1 μm) is commonly used in radiography. Besides silver halide and gelatin, the emulsion layer contains various additives like chemical sensitizers, wetting agents, antifoggants, hardeners, etc., which gives the required qualities to the film. The silver halide grains are typically 1–1.5 μm in diameter and contain 10^6–10^7 silver atoms. There are about 10^9 grains per cubic centimeter. Approximately four light photons must be absorbed to sensitize each grain.

Among the silver halides (AgBr, AgCl, AgI), silver bromide (AgBr) is the most used in film emulsion and its spectrogram is shown in Figure 3.2.

The formation of crystals is done in dark as follows; the metallic silver is dissolved in nitric acid, to form silver nitrate. This is mixed with potassium bromide, to form silver bromide. It is done in the presence of gelatin under given temperature and pressure conditions. The arrangement of atoms in the crystal are cubic and lattice structure, and has imperfections. These imperfections provide sensitivity centers, for latent image formation. Direct exposure film has thicker crystals than screen type film. The film speed is controlled by size and concentration of the crystal.

When the film is exposed to X-rays, photon interacts with bromine (photon + Br = Br + e⁻) and release secondary electrons (Figs. 3.3A to F). These interactions are either *photoelectric absorption* or *Compton scattering* type. These electrons migrate to the sensitivity center and get trapped. Mobile silver atoms (Ag⁺) are attracted to the sensitivity center, where

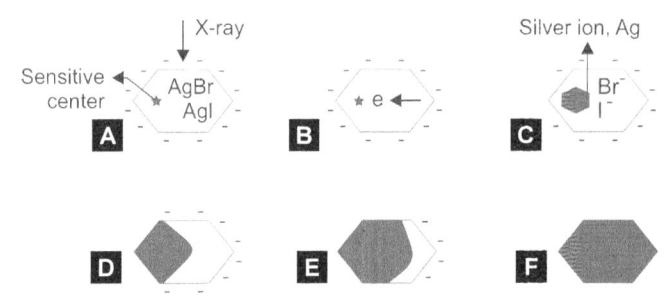

Figs. 3.3A to F: Latent image formation: (A) X-ray exposure provides electrons; (B) Electrons move to the sensitive center; (C) Mobile silver atoms move to the sensitivity center, combine with electron and form latent image; (D) Process repeated, latent image widens; (E) Additional silver formation during processing; and (F) Final metallic silver image.

they combine with electrons and become metallic silver ($Ag^+ + e^- = Ag$). These metallic silver atoms give latent image, which is invisible. Basically, the bromine and iodine are present at the surface, whereas silver is inside the crystal. Mostly electrons are provided by bromine and iodine atoms, resulting in collapse of crystal structure. As a result, bromine and iodine are free to move to the gelatin area. No more ionic force is acting in the crystal.

Overcoat

The gelatin is covered by a protective layer called overcoat or topcoat. It protects the light sensitive emulsion layer from scratches, pressure, contamination, and handling damages.

The X-ray film is duplitized, which means that all the above mentioned four layers are coated on both sides of the film. This helps in providing better density and contrast and also to reduce the exposure required. It also helps to avoid curling of the film. The thickness of a radiographic film ranges from 200 µm to 300 µm (0.25 mm).

FILM TECHNOLOGY

Gelatin

Initially collodion was used as substratum which was a mixture of *guncotton, ether* and *alcohol*. Some of the workers using collodion become addicted to the ether and alcohol vapor. Hence, it was replaced with gelatine about 100 years ago. Gelatin is a common protein, obtained from cartilage, skin, and ossein (protein matrix of bone). Collagen is converted into gelatin by the process known as *hydrolysis*. During this process, the water destroys the cross-linking of collagen and produces the gelatin polymer. The gelatin has the following properties:

- It absorbs the water present in processing and allows easy penetration of processing solutions.
- It reduces the amount of grain clumping by keeping individual crystals separate.
- It binds the emulsion to the film base.
- It provides a growth medium for silver halide, during manufacturing.
- It provides impurities of sulfur which give active points of silver sulfide. These points deepen electron traps and consume certain photo by-products.
- It allows production of electron traps, which are vital for latent image formation.
- It also prevents the recombination of bromide ions after their release by radiation exposure, so that it reduces latent image fade.

Silver Halides

The principal material in use is silver halide. These are metallic crystalline solids formed by reacting a suitable silver compound with one of the elements of halogen. The three useful halides are:
- Silver bromide (AgBr)
- Silver iodide (AgI)
- Silver chloride (AgCl).

All the three have a natural spectral sensitivity at *480 nm* (blue). Silver bromide is mostly used in emulsion manufacturing. It has a cut-off sensitivity at 480 nm and a peak sensitivity at *430 nm* (Fig. 3.4).

Silver chloride has a low inherent sensitivity, compared to silver bromide. However, it has an advantage in certain applications, in which it possesses very rapid development and fixing properties. Silver iodide

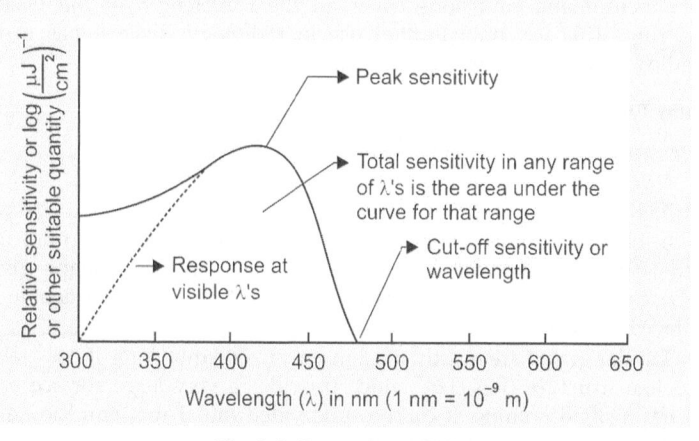

Fig. 3.4: Spectral sensitivity.

is only used in combination with either silver bromide or silver chloride. Usually, 2–4% of AgI is mixed with silver bromide for the manufacturing of X-ray emulsions. This increases its sensitivity and also extends its spectral response. The main disadvantages of AgI are:
O   Fixing time increases
O   It cannot be used independently.

Spectral Sensitivity

The spectral sensitivity of the emulsion is the range of wavelengths of the electromagnetic spectrum to which the emulsion will respond. It is usually plotted wavelength versus relative sensitivity as *spectrogram*. Peak sensitivity is the wavelength in which the emulsion exhibits its highest response. The cut-off sensitivity is the wavelength beyond which the film is no longer sensitive (*see* Fig. 3.4). Extending the natural sensitivity of the silver halides is called *spectral sensitizing*. This can be achieved by adding a suitable dye to the emulsion. The spectral sensitivity of film emulsion can be divided into three categories, namely:
O   Monochromatic emulsions
O   Orthochromatic emulsions
O   Panchromatic emulsions.

Monochromatic emulsions are blue sensitive and non-color sensitive. It is often called as blind emulsion, meaning that it cannot see any colors of longer wavelength than blue. It is mostly used in X-ray imaging.

Orthochromatic emulsions are those, that have a spectral sensitivity up to and including green part of the visible spectrum. This can be further classified as short, medium, and long orthochromatic emulsions. These films are used with rare-earth screens (green) and in monitor photography, etc.

Panchromatic emulsions cover all the wavelength of the visible spectrum. This has only limited use in radiology, since it has to be handled in complete darkness during processing.

Grain Types

There are two types of grains, namely:
O   Globular grain
O   Tabular grain.

In blue sensitive or monochromatic films, only globular grains are used (Fig. 3.5). Globular means spherical and spherical shape gives highest volume, which provides good absorption. This will enable to achieve higher speed.

Tabular grains are mostly used in sensitized emulsions. It has "table top" like structure (Fig. 3.6), which provides a very large surface area but has a small volume. It can be subdivided into T-mat emulsion and structured twins. *T- mat* is a trademark of **Kodak** limited, in which all

Medical X-ray Film

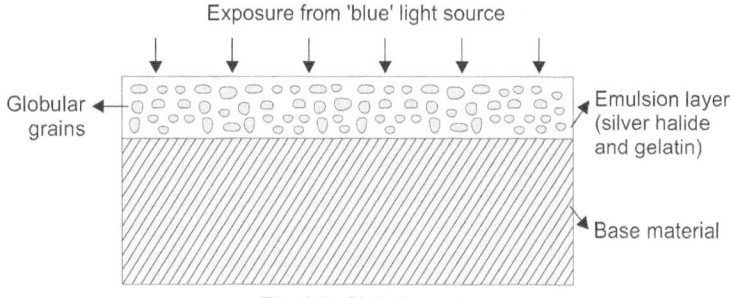

Fig. 3.5: Globular grain.

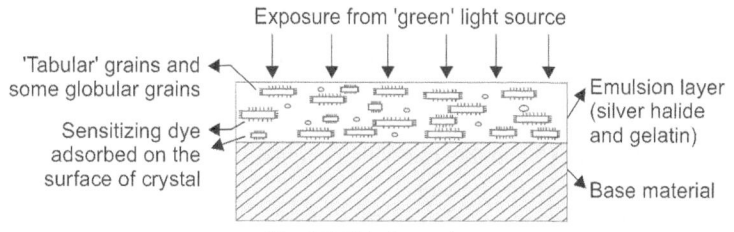

Fig. 3.6: Tabular grain.

grains are identical and extremely flat. *Structured twins* is a trademark of **Agfa-Gevaert** Limited. In this, the surface area of the crystal is achieved by using two tabular type grains in combination. The advantages of tabular grains are:
- Increased resolution
- Reduction in silver weight (thin crystal)
- Less processing time.

FILM TYPE, SIZE, AND PACKING

Film Types

Basically all the imaging films are divided into two categories:
- *Screen type*:
  - Single side coated
  - Double side coated
- Direct exposure type.

Screen Type Film

Screen type film, which is also called as duplitized film is more sensitive to light. When this film is used with intensifying screens, it is faster than the direct exposure film. Screen type films are generally used in radiography.

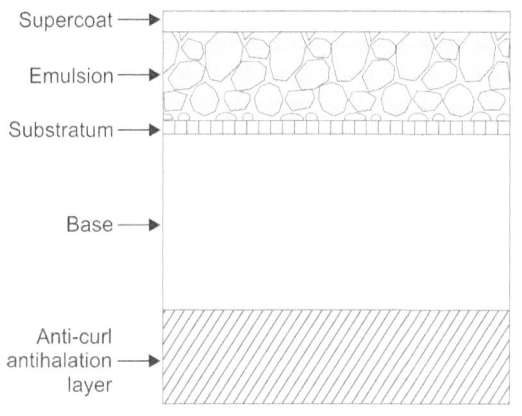

Fig. 3.7: Single-coated film.

The advantage of screen type film is that it increases the sensitivity of the system, which may have the following benefits:
- Reduces dose to the patient
- Reduces movement unsharpness
- Reduces geometric unsharpness
- Reduces dose to hospital staff.

Single-coated films have an emulsion layer on only one side of the film base (Fig. 3.7), whereas double-coated films have two emulsion layers. Invariably different types of emulsions are used. These films are provided with *anti-curl backing* and *anti-halation layer*. Anti-curl backing prevents the film curling during processing and allows the film to stay flat after processing. For this purpose, another layer of gelatin is coated on the non-emulsion side. Anti-halation layer is a colored dye included in the gelatin of anti-curl backing. *Halation* is caused by the reflection of light at the boundary of the base with the air. This reduces halo unsharpness effect that reduces resolution. The dyes used in antihalo layers are designed to absorb light that passes through the base and into the anti-curl/halation layer. Screen-film selection depends on the following:
- Contrast
- Speed
- Spectral matching
- Crossover
- Safe light.

It is available with low- and high-contrast levels and multiple latitudes. High-contrast film contains uniform and smaller size grains and produces black and white image. Low-contrast film have large grains with wide range of sizes and gives gray image. Films are available with different speed, and it is controlled by grain size and shape. Screen type film has double side emulsion with double the speed of single side emulsion film. In general, speed refers for a combination of film and two screens. The proper matching of film and screen is required for speed accuracy.

The light from a given screen may expose the base on the opposite emulsion, which is called *crossover*. Tabular grains reduce crossover significantly. Crossover can be minimized by:
O   Adding a light absorbing dye
O   Intensifying screens that emits shorter wavelengths (blue or UV).

Introduction of *rare-earth screens* require proper spectral matching. The rare-earth screens emit UV, blue, green, and *red light*. The film is sensitive to blue and violet not for green and red. Hence, the film is spectrally sensitized with special types of dyes. If green emitting screen is used, the film should be sensitive to blue and green light. This is called spectral matching and the film is called green sensitive film or orthochromatic film. If there is mismatching, it will reduce the speed and give higher patient dose.

Safe light provides illumination in the dark room, keeping the film unexposed. A 15 watt bulb at 1.5 m from the work bench is the correct choice. For a blue sensitive film an amber light (550 nm) is used. This light will fog the green sensitive film. Therefore, a red filter (660 nm) should be used for green sensitive film. Red filter can be used for both blue and green sensitive film.

Direct Exposure Film

The emulsion of a direct exposure film is thicker and consists of high concentration of AgBr crystals, with single side emulsion. They are mainly used to image thinner body parts such as hands, feet, etc. It employs higher radiographic techniques and offer increased radiation dose to the patient. It is rarely used today in medical imaging.

Direct exposure films are sensitive to the direct action of X-rays. It is four times faster than screen film and its emulsion size is thicker. These films have the following special features:
O   Higher resolution
O   Higher silver coating weight
O   Lower speed
O   Maximum high density
O   Higher contrast
O   Dental film is an example for direct exposure type.

Dental Film

Dental films are used for two applications, namely; *intraoral* and *extraoral* view. Intraoral films are double emulsion films, direct exposure type and are available in 5.7 cm × 7.6 cm, 3.1 cm × 4.1 cm, and 2.2 cm × 3.5 cm sizes. Intraoral films are made with an outer packet or wrapper, which

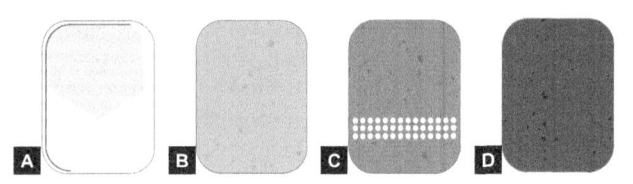

Figs. 3.8A to D: Dental film: (A) The outer wrapper; (B) The film; (C) The lead foil sheet; (D) The protective black paper.

is a waterproof paper or plastic. It is sealed to prevent the ingress of saliva. The side of the packet that faces toward the X-ray beam has either a pebbled or a smooth surface and usually white. The reverse side is usually of two colors, to avoid wrong placement of film in the mouth. The black paper on either side of the film is to protect from light, saliva, and damage by fingers. There is a lead foil on the back side of the film, to prevent the following:

- Residual radiation passing through the film to patient's tissues
- Back scattered radiation, comes from the tissues to film, which will degrade the final image.

The lead sheet also contains an embossed pattern to ensure correct placement. When the film is placed in a wrong way, the pattern will appear on the radiograph. There is a raised dot on the dental film to denote the tube side, after the film has been processed (Figs. 3.8A to D). Some manufacturers pack two films together to enable two films to be produced from one exposure. This film can be exposed without screen. This film has application as *periapical, bitewing,* and *occlusal* radiography.

Extraoral films are available either with non screen or with screen. Non screen film emulsion thickness is greater and requires long exposure time. The other type of dental film is an indirect action film or screen type film. These films are used in the following X-ray examinations:

- Panoramic view
- Oblique lateral view
- Skull view
- Intraoral vertex occlusal radiography.

These films are similar in design as general radiography films. Films with different emulsions are available in the market, which are sensitive to different colors of light, emitted by different screens. It is essential that the correct combination of film and intensifying screens should be used.

Overall, the various types of films used in dental radiography can be classified as follows:

- *Intraoral*:
    - Periapical film
    - Bite wing film
    - Occlusal film

○ *Extraoral*:
- ❏ Withscreen
- ❏ Nonscreen

Mammography Film

Mammography film is a single side emulsion type orthochromatic film, and is used with single intensifying screen at the back side. It uses both split emulsion layer and the cubic crystal technology. It provides two emulsion layers on one side of the film. Each layer consists of mono dispersed cubic silver crystal of identical size. The first layer provides high contrast in breast parenchyma and improved visualization. The second layer provides maximum density to visualize radio dense breast. In addition, it provides increased gradient and high dynamic range. Nowadays, green emitting *terbium-doped gadolinium oxysulfide* screens with green sensitive film is used. It offers superior image quality with reduction of radiation dose up to 40%. The surface of the film base opposite the screen is coated with a light absorbing dye, to reduce reflection of light from the screen. The above coating is called *anti-halation* coating and the effect is called halation. This coating is removed during processing, to improve image viewing.

Laser Film

Laser films are used in computed tomography, magnetic resonance imaging, and computed or digital radiography. Basically, digital electronic signal from the imaging system modulates a laser signal, proportional to the image signal. The laser beam writes the image on the film in raster fashion. The film is a silver halide film that has been sensitized to red light, which is emitted by the laser. Laser printers are light sensitive and hence, require darkness for operation. Different types of lasers are used and offer consistent image quality. It is also available with multiple film sizes and multiple image formats per film.

Specialty Film

Specialty film includes cine films used in angiography and spot films used in fluoroscopy imaging. Cine film is 35 mm width and is supplied in rolls of 100 ft and 500 ft. Spot films are 70–105 mm width and are used in cameras. They are similar to cine film, but larger in size, and can be viewed directly. Processing is very critical in the above types of films and requires special processors. It has single side emulsion and is provided with small notch in one corner of the film. Due to digitization of imaging equipment, the use of above films is declining today.

Film Size and Packing

Films are available in variety of sizes and packing. The common sizes are:

- 17″ × 17″, 17″ × 14″,
- 15″ × 12″, 15″ × 6″,
- 14″ × 14″, 14″ × 11″,
- 12″ × 12″, 12″ × 10″, 12″ × 6″,
- 10″ × 8″,
- 8.5″ × 6.5″,
- 6.5″ × 4.5″ (all dimensions are in inches).

Film is usually supplied in boxes of 25, 50, 100, and 500 sheets, with *folder wrapped* (FW) or *alternate folder wrapped* (AFW) as shown in Figure 3.9. In the FW packing each sheet of film is individually wrapped in a folded sheet of photographic quality paper. This will reduce abrasion marks on the surface of the film. This may occur as the films rub against each other during transportation, removal from the film hopper and during loading into the cassette. It also protects against finger marking, while handling. In the AFW packing every other film in the box has its own separate cover of paper. The paper used must be pure and free from any contamination.

Apart from this, *non-interleaved film* (NIF) packing is also possible. In this, the film is not protected from its neighbours, which is due to the following:
- Hardening of the super coat
- Hermetically sealed vacuum packs of plastic.

These packs hold the sheets firmly together, eliminating movement between adjacent sheets. These plastic packs are further placed in a strong outer box of high quality card, so that they are protected from humidity and chemical fumes. These cardboard cartons are labeled with identification mark of batch number and expiry date.

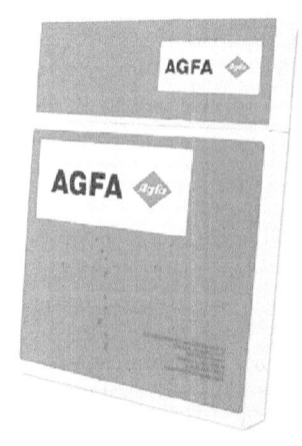

Fig. 3.9: Typical X-ray film box, containing 100 films per box. (*Courtesy*: M/s. Agfa Healthcare India Pvt Ltd)

CHARACTERISTICS OF X-RAY FILM

The characteristics of an X-ray film can be discussed with the following parameters:
○ Density
○ Characteristic curve
○ Contrast
○ Latitude
○ Emulsion absorption.

Density

The term density refers to the degree of blackening on the film. When the film is exposed to X-rays, the metallic silver gives the blackness on the film. That is why X-ray film is said to be a negative recorder. The degree of blackness is directly related to the intensity of radiation exposure. It can be quantified by a term *optical density* (OD), which is given by the relation:

$$OD = \log_{10} (I_0/I_t)$$

where, (I_0/I_t) is the inverse of transmittance (T), which is measured by a densitometer. If I_0 is the light intensity measured without film and I_t is the light transmitted through the film, then $T = I_t/I_0$. The useful range of density in diagnostic radiology is 0.25–2.0. As OD increases, the transmittance decreases.

Characteristic Curve

The relation between radiation exposure and OD is plotted as a curve, known as the characteristic curve or H and D curve, named after **Hurter** and **Driffield**, who first generated these curves in 1890. The film density is plotted on the vertical axis and log of film exposure on the horizontal axis (Fig. 3.10). The curve has sigmoid shape and has three portions, namely:
○ Toe
○ Straight line
○ Shoulder.

The toe is the low exposure region, and the shoulder is the high exposure region of the curve. *Base plus fog* level is the film blackening in the absence of any radiation exposure and typically ranges from 0.1 to 0.25 OD units. It refers the background fogging and the tinting (blue) of the base. The maximum film density ranges from 2.5 to 3.0 OD units.

All radiographic techniques should produce a density in the straight line portion. The contrast is related to the slope of the linear portion of the curve. Higher the slope, higher is the image contrast. The parameter which describes the contrast of the film is called *average gradient* or *film gamma*. It is the slope of the straight line portion, connecting two given points in the characteristic curve:

Medical X-ray Film Processing

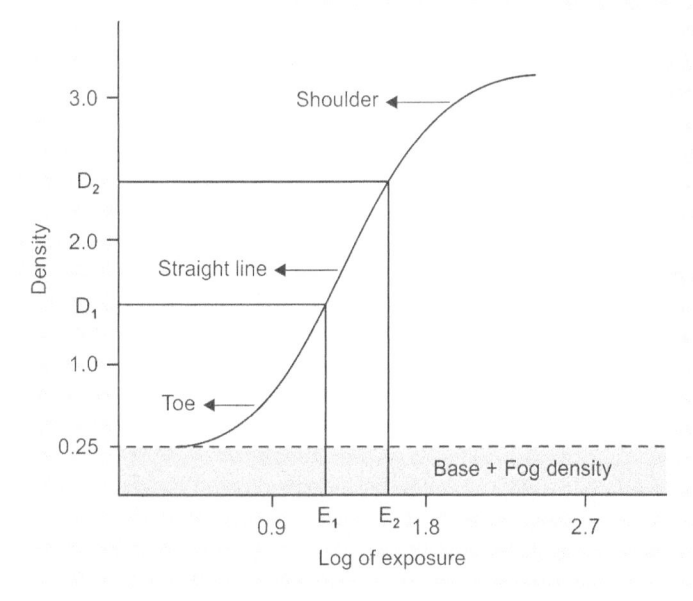

Fig. 3.10: Characteristic curve of the X-ray film.

$$\text{Average gradient} = \frac{(D_2 - D_1)}{\log_{10}(E_2 - E_1)}$$

where, D_2 and D_1 are the optical densities on the straight line portion of the curve, resulting from log of exposure E_2 and E_1. The average gradient value ranges from 2.5 to 3.5. The gradient is the mean slope between two specified densities. A high gradient refers higher radiographic contrast of the film.

Speed

The speed refers the sensitivity of the film-screen combination. Fast film requires lesser radiation exposure to achieve a given film density and slow film requires more radiation exposure. There are two types of speed in use, one is the *absolute speed* and the other is the *relative speed*. The absolute speed of a film is defined as the reciprocal of the exposure in roentgens (1/R) that required to produce a density of 1.0, above the base plus fog density. It is determined from the H and D curve and is used only in performance evaluation.

The relative speed is a measure, compared with a standard film screen-film combination. For example, *calcium tungstate* screen-film combination is called *par speed* and given a value of 100. Any other combination of screen-film having twice the speed of calcium tungstate is given the speed of 200. In this way the rare-earth screen combination is given speed of 400, which is used in general radiography. Angiograms involve short exposures, may require a speed of 600. Bone and extremities require more detail or slow films.

Latitude

Latitude is the range of exposure levels (mAs) that will produce acceptable range of density (0.25–2.0). The latitude is also called dynamic range, varies inversely with film contrast. A wide latitude film has a shallow gradient and low contrast, whereas short latitude films will have high gradient and higher contrast (Fig. 3.11). A technologist may have more freedom in wide latitude films, so that he can select the desired exposure technique. However, it is prone for errors, which are difficult to understand. On the other hand, in a short latitude film, the exposure is limited and more critical. Even a slight change in exposure may increase the contrast manifold. Hence, a proper balance has to be made between contrast and latitude. A low-latitude film may require number of retakes, because exact exposure techniques are difficult to decide.

Contrast

The contrast is the density difference between two adjacent image areas in a radiograph. The film contrast tells us how the film responds to the difference in exposure. The film contrast depends on the following factors:
○ Characteristic curve
○ Film density
○ Screen or nonscreen exposure
○ Film processing.

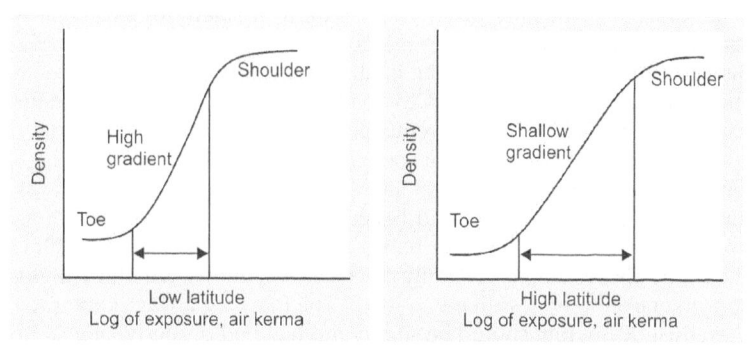

Fig. 3.11: Comaprison of low latitude and high latitude films: Low latitude gives high contrast, whereas high latitude film gives low contrast.

Film contrast is determined by the slope of the characteristic curve. The film gamma is the maximum slope of the characteristic curve. Double emulsion films produce greater contrast than single emulsion films. High-contrast single emulsion films are used in mammography.

Emulsion Absorption

It is necessary that silver halide grains in the film must absorb the light emitted by the intensifying screen. The ability of silver halide to absorb light depends on the wavelength or color of light. Generally, silver halide absorbs light in the UV, violet, and blue regions. It is possible to expand the sensitivity of the film to green color with a coating of dye. Such green sensitive film is called *orthofilm*. The silver halide, coated with a dye which absorbs red light is called *pan film*.

FILM HANDLING AND STORAGE

X-ray film is a delicate material and it should be handled carefully. The film should be handled always only by its edges with clean and dry hands. One should avoid touching the film surfaces. Do not touch the film surface with finger nails, scissors, knives, and screw drivers. When handling the film in the processing room, all white light is switched off. The film should be handled either in darkness or under safe light. Film should be exposed to the safe light lamp for a period equal to unload a film from the cassette. Films left out under safe light lamp, for too long will fog. If the film cannot be processed at once, it should be stored in a light-tight container.

When loading films in hangers for development, they should be protected from direct light from lamp. Improper safe light illumination is a common cause of film fog. Excessive examination of films under safe light causes *aerial fog* on films. The illumination will be safe only, if bulbs of less than 15 watts are used. The standard of safety for safe light is such that, unexposed X-ray film may be safely handled in the light of a distance of 3 ft for 1 minute. The loading bench in the processing room should be grounded, so that in the handling of the cassette, any static charge that are built up can be removed before the cassette is opened.

X-ray film must be stored at cool places, both day and night. At high temperatures, the film will be spoiled before the expiry date. The X-ray film is sensitive to pressure and hence, it should be kept always in an upright (vertical) position like books on a bookshelf. Therefore, films should be always stored vertically on the edges. In this, the film will not stick to one another, less likely to wrap. The films are always kept away from dust. X-ray film should be stored and handled properly, otherwise it will produce artifacts. It should not be bent, creased, or rough handled. It is pressure-sensitive, and sharp objects like finger nails may produce artifact. Film is sensitive to temperature and humidity, and should be stored at 20°C. Higher temperature and humidity (>60%) may cause fog and reduce image contrast.

Film is sensitive to light and should be stored and handled in dark. Exposure to low level light may increase the fog. Hence, a well-sealed dark room and a lightproof storage bin is a must. Ionizing radiations may fog the film and reduce contrast. Film is more sensitive after an exposure than before. In the first exposure the OD is raised above the toe. Successive exposure may cause higher OD. Film should not be stored near radioactive substance and nuclear medicine areas.

Films are supplied in boxes of 50 or 100 sheets. The packing may be by interleaved or noninterleaved method with chemically treated paper. Expiry date is given on the box, which is the *shelf life* of the film. Film should not be used after the expiry date, which is usually 6 months. Aged films may have loss of speed, contrast with increased amount of fog. The storage is made in such a way that oldest film should be used first. Film may be purchased monthly, so that the storage may not exceed more than 30 days.

4
Darkroom, Cassette, and Intensifying Screens

DARKROOM

The darkroom is a film processing room. It must be located adjacent to the X-ray room or central to the X-ray rooms. The common wall will have a hatch, to pass cassettes to the darkroom. This will not only save time but also wear and tear of the cassette. It must have sufficient space, about 10′ × 10′ × 10′ (cubic feet). The walls of the darkroom must be thick enough (25/35 cm) to protect against scattered/primary radiation. The floor should be durable, easily cleaned, not slippery, and resistant to staining and corrosive substances. Windows should be avoided and air conditioning is the ideal choice.

A red light at the entrance to the darkroom is essential, so that it will indicate that the work is in progress inside. Everything must be done to ensure that no light from outside can penetrate into the darkroom, even when anyone enters or leaves it. The entrance of the darkroom must be light-tight and is provided with interlocked doors. In order to prevent electrical shock, all metallic objects must be earthed. The ideal darkroom installation is shown in Figures 4.1A and B. It mainly consists of the following:

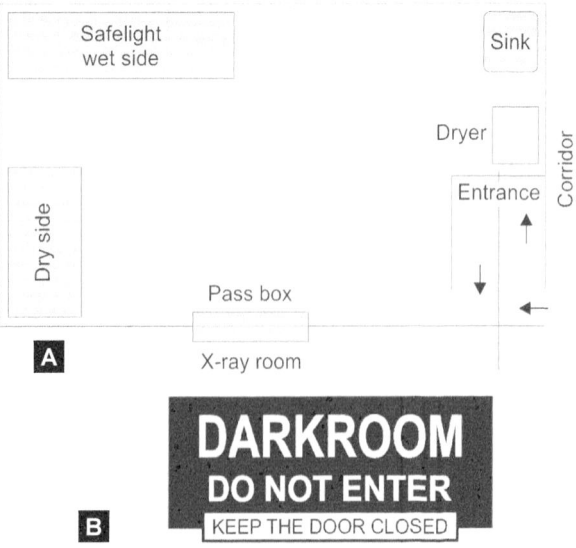

Figs. 4.1A and B: (A) An ideal darkroom; (B) Darkroom placard at the entrance.

- Dry side
- Wet side
- Safelight
- Pass box.

There are three possible systems for ensuring safe access to a darkroom.

1. *Double door entrance*: Two doors placed one behind the other, with enough space between them to allow one person to enter and close the outer door before opening the inner one (Fig. 4.2A). In order to prevent one of the two doors from being left slightly open by someone in a hurry, a bell or buzzer is installed which continues to ring as long as one of the doors is open. There are also mechanical or electrical systems ensuring that it is impossible to open one door as long as the other is not completely closed. A defect in such a system may mean that someone has to spend a short while imprisoned in the lock. Its advantage is space economy.

2. *Labyrinth or maze*: The labyrinth type entrance is by far best solution, but it is more space-consuming (Fig. 4.2B). The sidewalls of a labyrinth entrance are black, in order to exclude any reflected light. A white strip, approximately 4-inch wide, runs at about 5 feet from the ground along all the walls of the labyrinth, and serves as a completely clear signpost.

3. *Revolving door*: This system is good and looks simpler. This means, all possibilities of error are excluded. This is similar to the gate in a park or hotel, which allows only one person at a time, in the shape of X. When a person is in a very great hurry, it is still not the ideal system. This system has the advantage of not taking up too much space, but not common in practice.

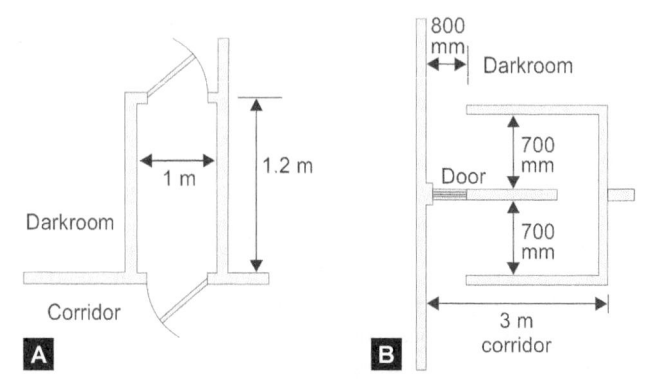

Figs. 4.2A and B: Various types of entrances: (A) Double doors; (B) Labyrinth entrance.

Walls, Floor, and Ceiling

The inside walls of the darkroom are light colored. This is for psychological reasons, since black walls are very depressing in their effect. The darkroom light must be easily reflected by the walls, while film processing. Also black color induces the feeling of "no space", which causes an unpleasant impression. A glossy cream or white paint on the walls would serve the purpose, since they reflect the safe lamp light adequately. Glazed tile walls are to be recommended, from point of view of upkeep. They can be washed regularly with water, and this is necessary in order to combat dust, which is great enemy to the darkroom.

The type of paint on the ceiling is important, because it will produce flakes, which are likely to fall on the film/cassette. Hence, plaster is to be avoided. A good quality, modern emulsion paint is satisfactory. To avoid similar risk of falling particles, water pipes, electric conduits or air ducts should be enclosed above a false ceiling. The choice of floor material should adhere the following conditions:

- It is nonporous
- It is resistant to staining by chemicals/liquids
- It does not become slippery when wet.

An absorbent floor covering cannot easily be cleaned. Material which has high proportion of asphalt is satisfactory (porcelain and natural clay tiles). Some varieties of hard rubber and rubber sheet will also serve the purpose. Adhesive material used to fasten down floor cover must be waterproof.

Dry Side

The darkroom is installed in two distinct parts namely, the dry side and the wet side. This separation is very much essential and need to be respected at all times. A darkroom assistant, by constant practice, can adapt this separation as a natural one. Any wet objects and chemicals are to be excluded from the dry side, so that it is dry always. It is here that the cassettes are loaded and emptied. Even a slightest drop of water or chemical solution can cause defects on the film.

The dry side is provided with a dry loading bench, which is covered with a sheet of fiber-board, linoleum or plastic material. The dimension of the dry bench is such that, it is long enough to allow 3 or 4 of largest cassettes to be placed upon it side-by-side without an overlap, when they are opened. The recommended length and width is 2.5 m and 0.6 m per operator. The height should not be less than 0.9 m; preferably mounted on a plinth, to allow toe space. The bench is equipped as follows:

- A set of pigeon-holes for unopened boxes.
- A light-tight, folding sectional box for films with an electrical safety device.

Darkroom, Cassette, and Intensifying Screens

- A store place for cassettes.
- A closed waste-paper basket for package and interleaving paper, etc.
- One or several drawers for all kinds of accessories (scissors, clips, writing and marking material, rubber stamps, safelight lamps/filters, thermometer, etc.).

The film hangers should not be suspended over the center of the dry loading bench. If they fell accidentally, they will damage the films or the intensifying screens. Film hangers should be placed on special hooks which are fixed into the sidewall on the dry side.

Wet Side

The wet side is a place where the film is chemically processed and finally becomes a radiograph. The wet side consists of the following items:
- Processing chemicals
- Two stirring paddlers
- Thermometer
- Stop clock
- Processing tanks.

In order to prevent electrical shock, all metallic objects must be earthed.

A series of tanks for the baths are placed next to each other, and they form a large built-in unit. This unit is available in the market in various sizes. An automatic temperature regulating device is necessary, to maintain the temperature. Two stirring paddlers are required to prepare developer and fixer solution.

The tanks may be made of stainless steel, plastic or hard rubber. Stainless steel tanks are preferable for normal darkroom use. The size of the tanks needs to be suitable for the maximum size of the films used and the number of films to be processed per hour. The space between the films in the bath has to be at least 0.8 inches. The upper edge of the film is approximately 1 inch below the level of the bath. In addition, there is a possibility of placing at least four films in the tank at one time. The wet side is equipped with at least four tanks, arranged in the order of processing:
- Developing tank
- Tank for rinsing
- Fixing bath
- Tank for washing (Fig. 4.3).

The simplest one consists of a three-compartment tank, meant for developing, rinsing/washing, and fixing. The middle compartment should be provided with running water. A fixing tank should have about twice the volume of a developing tank, since the fixing time is two times the developing time. The washing tank volume should be about twice the size of the fixing tank.

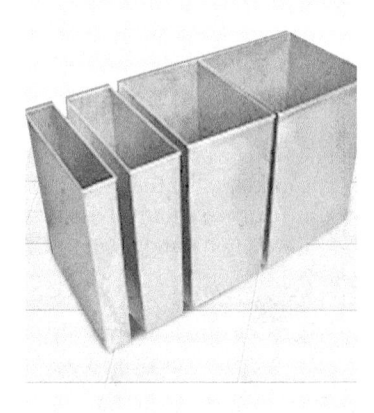

Fig. 4.3: Processing tanks for developer, rinsing, fixing and washing at the wet side of the darkroom.

Safelight

The darkroom is illuminated by a safelight, which will not fog films. A safelight is one which exerts very little effect on the X-ray film, so that the films can be handled without the risk of damage. It can be either *direct or indirect safelighting*. X-ray films are sensitive only to green, blue, and ultraviolet light. It is insensitive to certain portion of blue and green also. Usually, special monochromatic lamps such as green, orange, yellow, brown or red lamps of <25 W are used as safelights. Generally, brown or olive-green lighting is preferred. They emit a wavelength for which we have greater visual sensitivity at low level of illumination. In the case of direct safelight, a 15 W bulb is recommended. The working distance between the safelight and the film should not be less than 1.2 m. It may be reduced to 0.6 m, if a 15 W bulb is used.

In the case of indirect safelight, bulb wattage up to 25 W can be used. In this method, the safe lamp directs the light towards the ceiling which reflects it back into the room. One depends entirely on reflection from the walls and ceiling of the darkroom. One indirect light for every 6.5 m^2 of ceiling area, at a height of 2.1 m above floor level should be sufficient to provide a good illumination. Such safelights must be fitted with proper filters. Usually, a sheet of gelatin dyed to the approximate color, sandwiched between two sheets of glass. The glass also helps to diffuse light. The usefulness of safelight depends on the following parameters:

- Spectral sensitivity of the film
- Filter spectral transmission
- Bulb watts

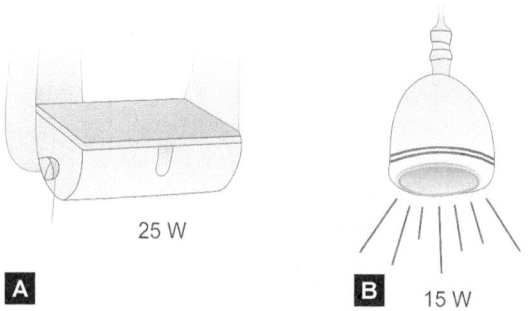

Figs. 4.4A and B: Safe light: (A) Indirect safelighting; (B) Direct safelighting.

- Exposure time
- Distance between the film and light.

The effectiveness of the safelight is tested periodically. It should be tested for a particular film type before it is used clinically. To do this, place a coin on an unexposed film. The film is exposed under safelight for 1 minute. It is repeated for 2, 3, 4, and 5 minutes and finally processed. Let us find the time in which the outline of the coin is just visible. This is the maximum time that the film can be left open under the safelight without fog. Films that are exposed to X-ray are more sensitive (8 times) to safelight. Hence, their handling-time must be as short as possible (<1/10 of the selected time in fog test). A typical safelight is shown in Figures 4.4A and B.

Pass Box

The darkroom is connected to the X-ray room by means of a pass box (Fig. 4.5). The cassette pass box is a small box built into an opening in the wall, provided with doors on each side. It has opening into the darkroom and into the X-ray room, respectively. It has two light-tight X-ray proof doors, which are revolving on vertical axis. The pass box is designed in such a way that no light from the X-ray room can penetrate into the darkroom. In most cases, a mechanical or electrical system is installed, so that it is impossible to open simultaneously both the doors. The pass box is divided into two compartments. One is for passing through the unexposed film-cassette and the other is for returning the exposed film-cassette.

Air-conditioning System

The room should be provided with air-conditioning, which is more efficient than cross ventilation by fans. Darkroom temperatures should be maintained at 18.3°C (65°F). The relative humidity of the atmosphere should be ideally 40–60%.

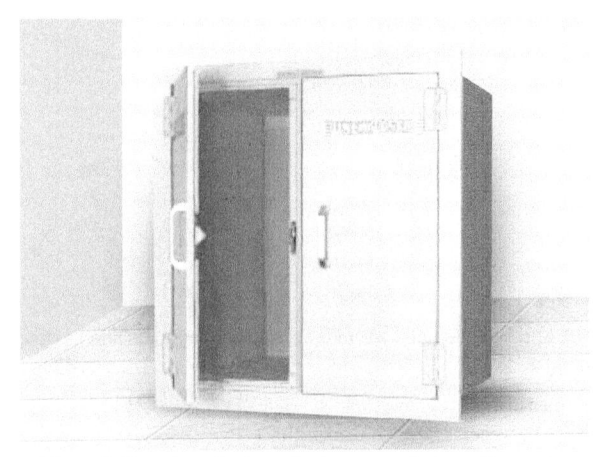

Fig. 4.5: Pass box for transferring cassette in radiography.

Maintenance

The darkroom needs day-to-day maintenance and good housekeeping. The developing and fixing solutions should be changed regularly, since they become weaker with use and age. These chemicals can damage skin and clothing, and hence, proper care is very much needed. In addition, one should adhere the following:
- Every day in the morning, the developer and fixer solutions should be stirred using the rods provided to them.
- These chemicals, tanks and rods should not be mixed and kept separately with labeling.
- The developing tank and fixing tank should be kept with full of developer and fixer solutions.
- The developer and fixer solution should be changed once in 30 days or lesser, depending upon the workload.
- The water in the rinsing/washing tank must be changed everyday. Running water should be preferred.
- The developer, fixer solutions, rinsing and washing water should be maintained at the same temperature. The water must be clean. If it is muddy or dirty, proper filter must be used. The filter should be cleaned every week.

CASSETTE

A cassette is a lightproof rigid holder that contains screens and film (Fig. 4.6A). The front side is made up of material of low atomic number, like plastic or carbon fiber. The X-rays pass through the entire cassette.

Darkroom, Cassette, and Intensifying Screens

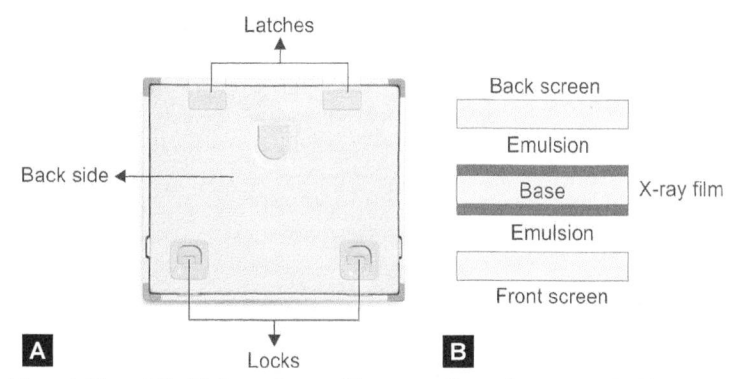

Figs. 4.6A and B: (A) Cassette used in screen-film radiography; (B) Placement of screens and film inside the cassette.

Some part of X-rays is backscattered from the back side of the cassette. This is known as *backscatter*, which results in image *fog*. Hence, the back side is usually made up of heavy metals (lead), having high atomic number, to minimize backscatter, which degrades image quality.

Inside the cassette, there are two permanently mounted intensifying screens, called front and back screens (Fig. 4.6B). The X-ray film is loaded between the two screens. The screens may have different thickness or equal thickness. Compressive materials such as felt or rubber is kept in between the screen and the cassette cover, at the back side. The compressive material maintains good screen-film contact, when the film is loaded. Cassettes are usually hinged on one side and can be opened from the other side. The film is loaded into the cassette in the darkroom. Cassettes are available in different sizes, namely:

- 8″ × 10″
- 10″ × 12″
- 14″ × 14″
- 14″ × 17″ (in inches).

Nowadays, *carbon-fiber* cassettes are available. The front side is made up of graphite fiber in a plastic matrix (carbon, Z = 6). It has 50% lesser absorption compared to aluminium or plastic. This will reduce patient radiation dose to a greater extent. That is why carbon-fiber cassette is preferred in pediatric radiology.

Loading the Cassette

When loading the cassette, it is opened like a book, or bring the lid upward on the top of the dry table. The intensifying screens, attached both inner side of the cassette, are now upward. A film and its folder are taken out of the film bin, using only the thumb and forefinger. If more fingers are used, it involves the risk of causing a crack in the film, leading to the appearance of a blackmoon-shaped mark on the film when it is

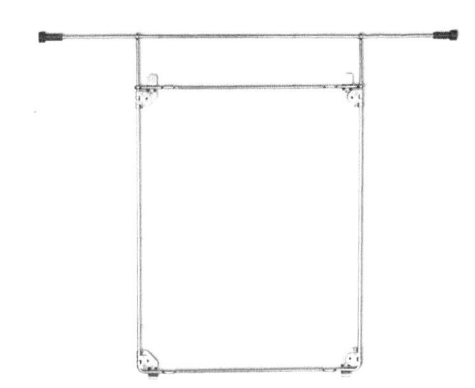

Fig. 4.7: X-ray film hanger.

developed. Continuing to hold the film in the same way, lift it up with the free hand on the underside, so that the lower part of the folder hangs down freely. In this way, the film is placed in the cassette and the folder is carefully removed, still being held in the right hand. After it has been shut and firmly locked, the cassette can be placed in the pass box. Now the cassette is ready for patient use and exposure.

Unloading the Cassette

Once the exposed film is back in the darkroom, the cassette is opened, and flipped back the compartment containing the film until the film falls out the edge against finger. It should be taken with two fingers only and fastened with the four corners of the clips of the hanger (Fig. 4.7) or slipped into the slot of the slide frame. The film is now ready for development, and it can be taken to the wet side of the darkroom.

INTENSIFYING SCREENSW

Film is insensitive to X-rays and requires more amount of X-rays to produce an image, which will increase patient dose. To avoid this, intensifying screens of about 200 μm thickness is used in cassettes in medical imaging. The film is sandwiched between two screens of equal thickness. This type of film is called double-emulsion film, which has emulsion on both sides. They absorb X-ray photons and emit more visible light or ultraviolet, for which the X-ray film is more sensitive. The light or UV exposes the film and gives the final image, which will improve the efficiency of radiographic imaging, with lesser patient dose. Thus, the intensifying screens amplify the effect of image formation with following advantages:

Darkroom, Cassette, and Intensifying Screens

- Shorter exposure time, resulting in lower patient dose
- Decrease in X-ray tube loading
- Decrease in motion blur.

Though it reduces patient dose, the image is slightly blurred. However, the image blur is not a series issue, nowadays with modern screen materials. Generally, intensifying screen consists of four layers, namely:
- Base
- Reflecting layer
- Phosphor
- Protective coat (Figs. 4.8A and B).

Base

The base is made up of *polyester* with 1 mm thickness. The base serves as a support on which the reflecting layer, phosphor, and protective layers

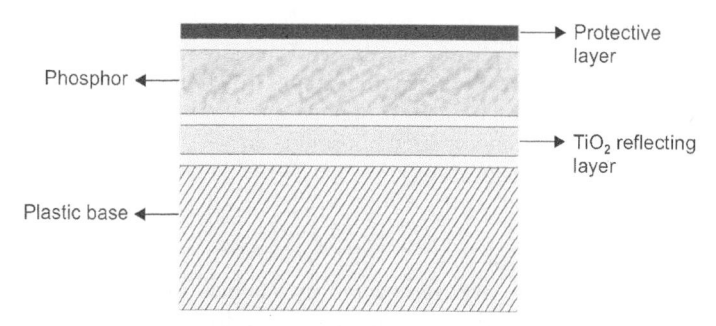

Fig. 4.8A: Intensifying screen.

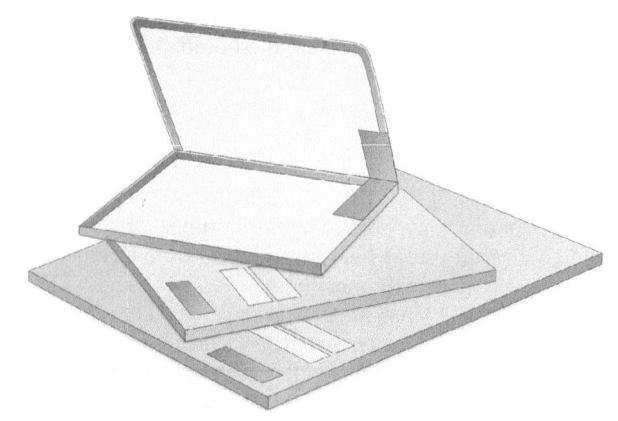

Fig. 4.8B: Commercial screen-film cassette, the part appears in white is the intensifying screens.
(*Courtesy*: M/s. Agfa Healthcare India Pvt. Ltd.)

are mounted. The base material should be moisture free, resistant to radiation damage and discoloration, chemically inert, and flexible.

Reflecting Layer

The reflecting layer is made up of by a white substance, such as *titanium dioxide* (TiO_2) or *magnesium oxide*. It is a shiny material of thickness 25 µm, which reflects light toward the phosphor and makes the light emission isotropic. Generally, half of the light is emitted towards the direction of the film and the rest is wasted. The reflecting layer redirects the light going in other directions towards the film. Thus, the reflective layer increases the efficiency of the intensifying screen, by doubling the number of light photons.

Phosphor

The phosphor is a crystal of inorganic salts, which emits light when exposed to X-rays. This is the backbone of the intensifying screen. The thickness of the phosphor ranges from 50 µm to 300 µm with individual crystal size of 5–15 µm. Generally, high atomic number material is used as phosphor. The commonly used phosphors are:
- Calcium tungstate ($CaWO_4$)
- Zinc sulfide
- Cesium iodide
- Barium lead sulfate.

Calcium tungstate was discovered by **Thomas A Edison** and was in use up to 1980, which emits blue light. The K-shell binding energy of tungsten is 69.5 keV, which is higher than the mean photon energy (40 keV) used in radiology. Hence, its K-edge absorption is lesser than optimal. Generally, phosphor material should have the following characteristics:
- It should have high atomic number, to have greater X-ray absorption.
- It should emit large amount of light per X-ray photon.
- The wavelength of light emitted should match the sensitivity of the X-ray film.
- The phosphor afterglow should be minimum.
- It should not be affected by heat, humidity, and environmental factors.

In recent times, rare earth phosphors (Z = 57–71) such as *gadolinium oxysulfide* ($Gd_2O_2S:Tb$), *lanthanum oxysulfide* ($La_2O_2S:Tb$), *lanthanum oxybromide* (*LaOBr*), *and yttrium tantalate* ($YTaO_4$) are used as screen phosphors. Gadolinium oxysulfide emits green light, whereas lanthanum oxybromide emits blue light. The light emitted by the screen should match the spectral sensitivity of the film, which is called *spectral matching*. Conventional film is sensitive to ultraviolet and blue light, whereas orthochromatic film is sensitive to green light.

The above screens can be manufactured with speed range of 200–1200. They have suitable K-shell absorption edges over the diagnostic photon energy of 35–70 keV. Their absorption and conversion efficiency is high. The spectral emission of rare earth phosphors is discrete and is centered at 540 nm. Therefore, green sensitive film must be used with these phosphors. These phosphors reduce patient dose, due to lower radiographic techniques. They also have less thermal stress and require lesser room shielding, as radiation levels are low. Though *cesium iodide* (CsI) is used in fluoroscopy and digital radiography, it is moisture sensitive and fragile. Hence, it is not used in screen-film radiography.

Protective Layer

The protective layer or coating (10–20 μm) is transparent to light and is facing the X-ray film. It is present at the top of the screen, so that it is resistant to abrasion and damage caused by handling. It also prevents formation of static electricity and provides a surface for cleaning. The total thickness of the intensifying screen is about 60 mg/cm^2.

Principle of Screen Function

When film alone is used, only 1% of the incident X-rays are absorbed, others (99%) get wasted. If screens are used with films, they absorb 50 times more than the films. When a part of X-rays pass through the front screen, the phosphor absorbs the X-rays and emits light in all directions. Every X-ray photon gives rise to hundreds of light photons. Thus, screen converts the X-ray pattern into a light pattern. The reflecting layer reflects the light toward the film, so that no photon is lost. Some portion of the X-rays that are bypassing through the X-ray film is absorbed and converted into light by the back screen. Thus, the intensifying screens convert large amount of X-ray photons (95%) into light photons of blue or green wavelength. Since the X-ray film is sensitive to blue or green light, it absorbs the entire light and gives the image (Fig. 4.9).

In the bottom picture there are 3 X-ray photons striking the screens at three different depths. Extreme right (C), the light photon travels longer path before reaching the film, resulting in greater light diffusion. The center beam (B) light photon travels lesser path and offer minimal light diffusion. Whereas the left side beam (A) travels moderate path and offers moderate light diffusion. Light diffusion causes screen blur and higher is the light diffusion, greater the screen blur. Intensifying screens decrease the exposure time and lower the patient dose.

The *absorption efficiency* of the screen refers to the percentage of X-ray photons absorbed in the screen. The *conversion efficiency* refers to how many light photons are produced by each absorbed X-ray.

68 Medical X-ray Film Processing

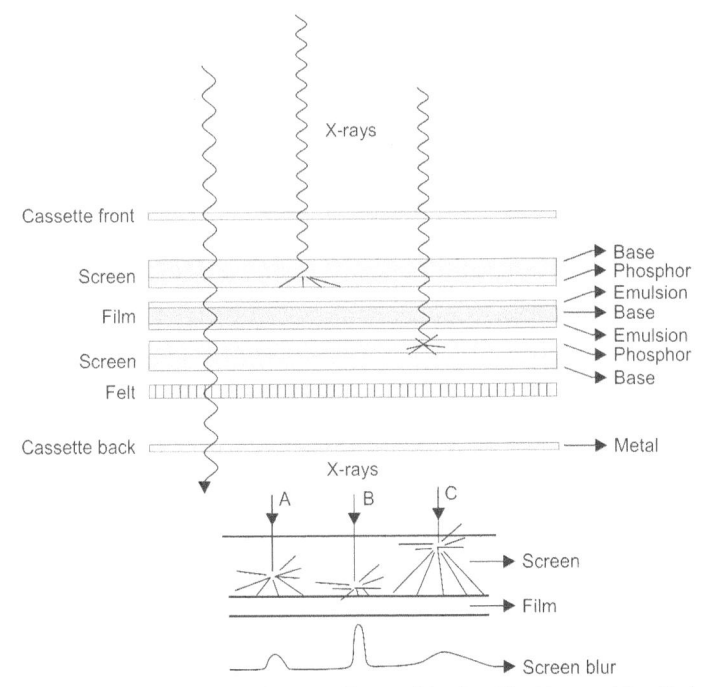

Fig. 4.9: Typical function of screen-film combination (double-emulsion film).

Screen Characteristics

Detective Quantum Efficiency

The detective quantum efficiency (DQE) or absorption efficiency of a screen is the ratio between amount of X-rays absorbed and amount of X-rays incident. Though thicker screens give higher DQE, they suffer with lateral light diffusion, resulting in blurred images. Thicker screen also reduces spatial resolution. This is the reason why two thin screens (both front and back) are used in radiography, which reduces the light diffusion path without loss of spatial resolution. The DQE of $Gd_2O_2S:Tb$ is highest for photon energy greater than 50 keV.

Conversion Efficiency

The conversion efficiency of a phosphor is the ratio between the amount of light emitted and the X-ray photons absorbed. It depends upon the intrinsic conversion efficiency of the phosphor. A 50 kV X-ray may emit about 5 keV light energy (10%). Usually, 1 keV light energy may consist of 500 light photons of each 2 eV energy. Conversion efficiency is 5% for calcium tungstate and 15% for $Gd_2O_2S:Tb$ with green light emission of wavelength of 545 nm. Presence of light absorbing dye reduces the conversion efficiency. The overall efficiency of screen-film system is the product of absorption efficiency and conversion efficiency.

Speed

The term speed is relative number, which describes how effectively X-rays are converted into light. The speed of a screen is inversely related to the *air kerma* (1/air kerma) required to produce a given density. As the speed increases, the air kerma required decreases. The air kerma values of fast (abdominal radiography), medium (chest radiography), slow (extremity radiography), and mammography screens are 2, 5, 20, and 200 µGy, respectively. The speed of a screen/film combination used in radiology ranges from 50 to 1,200, and is usually expressed relative to a standard screen. Calcium tungstate is referred as standard one with a speed of 100, known as *par-speed* screen.

Screen speed increases with screen thickness, absorption efficiency, and conversion efficiency. Screens are generally classified as fast, medium, and slow speed screens. High speed screens (1,200) are thicker and provide less spatial resolution with less patient exposure, e.g. rare earth screens. The rare earth screens are faster, because they have a higher absorption efficiency and higher conversion efficiency, at the mean X-ray energy used. Thicker screen increases image blur as a result of increased diffusion in the screen before striking the film. Slow speed screens (100) are thinner, but have better spatial resolution, e.g. detail screens. The various factors that influence the speed, image detail and patient radiation dose is given in Table 4.1.

Patient exposure is decreased greatly when intensifying screens are used. The reduction in patient exposure is measured by a term called *intensification factor* (IF). The IF is the ratio of the X-ray exposure needed to produce a given density (optical density of 1) on a film without screen and with the screen. It is a measure of speed of a screen, so that one can understand about the patient dose. The IF depends on the absorption and conversion efficiency of the screen. The usual intensification factors

Table 4.1: Relationship between screen speed, image detail and patient radiation dose for a given intensifying screen.

Parameter	Screen speed	Image detail	Patient radiation dose
Large crystal size	↑	↓	↓
Smaller crystal size	↓	↑	↑
Thicker phosphor	↑	↓	↓
Thinner phosphor	↓	↑	↑
Reflecting layer	↑	↓	↓
Absorbing layer	↓	↑	↑
Phosphor layer dye	↓	↑	↑

are 30–50. The Gd_2O_2S:Tb gives an intensification factor of 50, over the diagnostic X-ray range.

$$IF = \frac{\text{Exposure required without screen}}{\text{Exposure required with the screen}}$$

Generally, speed of the intensifying screens depends upon the following:
- Phosphor composition and thickness
- Crystal size and concentration
- Reflective layer
- Dye
- Kilo voltage
- Room temperature.

The first four factors are manufacture related and hence, called intrinsic factors. The last two are user-related and is called as an extrinsic factors. Rare earth phosphors with higher thickness increase speed. Reflective layer also increases speed, but also increases image blur. Dye decreases the speed, but improves spatial resolution. Larger crystal with higher concentration increases speed of the screen (Table 4.1). As the kV increases, the screen absorption decreases, resulting in increased intensification factors. Intensifying screens emit more light per X-ray photons at low temperatures, hence, the IF is higher. In other words, at higher temperature the IF is lower.

Noise

Noise appears on the radiograph as speckled background. It occurs when fast screens and high kVp techniques are used. In general, noise reduces image contrast. Screen with higher conversion efficiency increases noise. However, increase in absorption efficiency (DQE) will not affect the noise. Increase of conversion efficiency, enhances quantum mottle, resulting in higher noise. This may occur in very fast screens, with grainy and mottled image. Rare earth screens are two times faster than calcium tungstate, which do not increase noise significantly.

Spatial Resolution

Spatial resolution refers how small an object can be imaged and it is expressed in line pairs (lp) per millimeter. Higher is this number, better the spatial resolution, and smaller the object that can be imaged. X-ray test pattern is available to evaluate spatial resolution (Fig. 4.10). A typical test pattern consists of lead lines separated by spacers of equal thickness. The test tool is placed on the cassette with screen-film and exposed to X-rays. After developing the film, the lowest line pairs that is resolved is found. It gives the resolution of the screen-film combination. Contrast resolution is the ability to image similar body tissues, e.g. liver and pancreas. Spatial and contrast resolution are quantitative measurements that will jointly describe the image details.

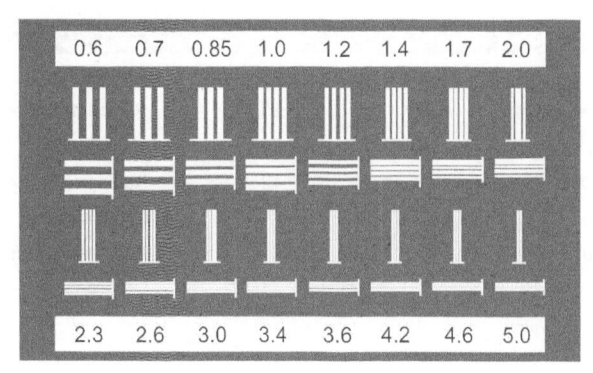

Fig. 4.10: Standard X-ray lead bar phantom for spatial resolution test: Group 16, Lead thickness 0.01–0.2 mm, test range: 0.6 lp/mm–5 lp/mm.

Screens have lower spatial resolution compared to direct exposure film. The spatial resolution is 7 lp/mm for fast screens, 15 lp/mm for fine-detail screen, and 50 lp/mm for direct exposure film. Human eye can resolve 10 lp/mm. When the film is used with screens, the light interacts with film by larger area, which is the cause for reduction in spatial resolution. Therefore, any increase in IF will always reduce spatial resolution. This is one of the reasons why screen is placed at the back side of the cassette in mammography. By doing so, the film is facing the tube side and thus, increases the spatial resolution. Smaller crystals and thinner phosphor layer always improves spatial resolution.

Screen-film Combination

Screen and film should have compatibility in order to produce quality images. In any screen/film combinations, the wavelength of light emitted by the screen and the sensitivity of the film must be matched (spectral matching). Generally, screen and film are specially designed for each other and always used in pairs. A proper screen-film combination gives the following advantages:
- Decrease of patient dose, occupational exposure, heat in X-ray tube, exposure time, mA and focal spot size
- Increase in kV selection flexibility, radiographic contrast adjustment, and special resolution.

Both front and back screen equally contribute to image formation. Rest 1% of the X-rays only directly interacts with film. Fast screen-film combinations are used for abdominal studies, whereas slow ones are used for extremity examinations. Dual screen, dual-emulsion systems are used in most cases. Single-emulsion, single screen systems are used for bone detail and mammography. The various screen characteristics and clinical applications are given in Table 4.2.

Medical X-ray Film Processing

Table 4.2: Various screens and clinical applications.

Screen	Composition	Resolution	Clinical use
Film alone	–	>25	Radiography (extremity)
Mammography	Gd_2O_2S: Tb	~20	Mammography
Detail (100)	La_2O_2S: Tb	~12	Radiography (extremity)
Par (400)	La_2O_2S: Tb	~7	Chest imaging
Fast (600)	$BaPbSO_4$	~5	Abdominal imaging

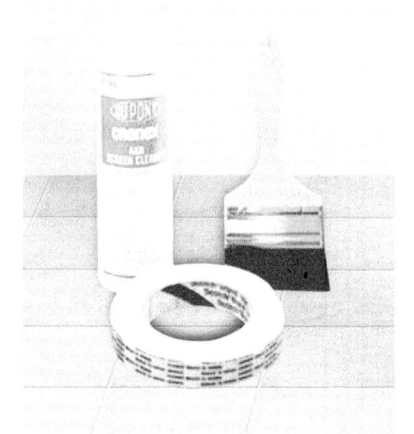

Fig. 4.11: Intensifying screen's cleaning solution for removing dirt, dust and finger prints, to increase screen life and efficiency.
(*Courtesy*: M/s. Agfa Healthcare India Pvt. Ltd.)

Handling and Care of Screens

Screen must be handled with care. Any foreign material on the screen, such as paper, blood, scratches, hair, dust, and stains will block light photons and produce area of underexposure, leading to artifact and image degradation. The film should not be made to slide into the cassette, while loading. Its sharp edge may scratch the screen. The film should be removed by tilting the cassette, so that the film fell down on the technologist hand. Finger nails should not be used to take the film from the cassette. The cassette should not be kept open in the dark room, to avoid damage by dust, etc.

The screen may be cleaned periodically (monthly) with a solution containing antistatic compounds or soap and water (Fig. 4.11). Further, it should be rinsed and dried after every cleaning. The frequency of

Darkroom, Cassette, and Intensifying Screens

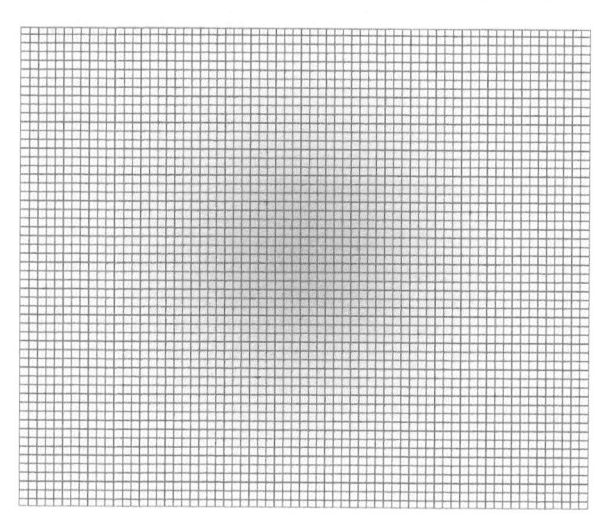

Fig. 4.12: Screen-film contact test by wire mesh pattern; poor contact shows blurred and cloudy pattern at the middle.

cleaning depends upon the use and level of dust in the environment. Film-screens should have good contact and this must be checked periodically with the help of a *wire mesh*. A poor screen-film contact will appear as blurred (block) and cloudy (Fig. 4.12). Such a cassette requires immediate replacement. This should be a part of regular quality control program. To ensure correct film density, nowadays *automatic exposure control* (AEC) is used. The AEC actually measures the incident radiation on the screen-film and terminates the exposure, after correct amount has been received.

5
X-ray Film Processing

MANUAL X-RAY FILM PROCESSING

Exposed X-ray films contain latent image which is invisible, since it has fewer silver ions that are converted into metallic silver. In processing, all the silver ions in the exposed crystal are converted to metallic silver. Later, the exposed crystal becomes black and the image is made visible. Thus, film processing converts the latent image into visible radiographic image. Film processing involves a series of organized procedures, namely:
- Development
- Rinsing
- Fixing
- Washing
- Drying (Fig. 5.1).

Development

Development is a chemical process that magnifies the invisible latent image into visible silver halide image. The solution used for this purpose is called *developer*. During the X-ray exposure, the $AgBr$ is divided into Ag^+ and Br^-. The developer converts the exposed silver ions into black metallic silver, by reduction process (addition of electron, $Ag^+ + e^- = Ag$).

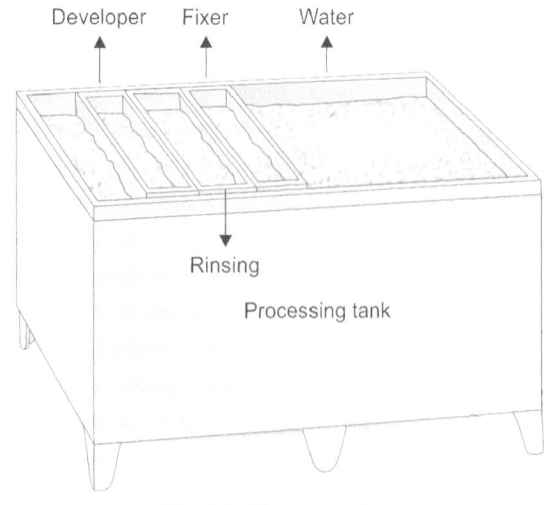

Fig. 5.1: Film processing.

X-ray Film Processing

The developer provides the electron to the sensitivity center and makes the silver atom neutral. This is why the developer is basically a *reducing agent*. The bromide negative ions, which are in the crystal lattice goes into the developer solution. The unexposed AgBr is unaffected by this process. An X-ray developer is basically an alkaline solution. There are two general types of developer solutions, namely:

- Regular X-ray developer
- Rapid X-ray developer.

The regular X-ray developer has average development potential. Its alkali is *sodium carbonate*. The rapid X-ray developer has high development potential. Its alkali is *sodium metaborate*. A developer solution contains the following composition:

- Developing agent
- Activator
- Restrainer
- Preservative
- Solvent.

Developing Agent

The purpose of a developing agent is to convert the exposed AgBr crystals into black metallic silver. This is called reduction process, and the chemical is known as *reducing agent*. In the reduction process, atom and molecules will gain electron. A good reducer is one which reacts more rapidly with exposed AgBr crystals only, than that are unexposed. At the same time it should also give a satisfactory image in a given development period at a given temperature. *Hydroquinone* plus *phenidone* or hydroquinone plus *metal* are used as developing agents. The former is 10–15 times more effective than the later. It is also less susceptible to the restraining effect of bromide concentration.

Hydroquinone is slow acting and is responsible for the high contrast (black shades). It is more sensitive to temperature. It works most efficiently when the solution temperature is less than 20°C. Phenidone is a reducing agent, acts rapidly and produces lighter gray shades. Phenidone controls the toe of the characteristic curve and hydroquinone controls the shoulder of the characteristic curve. Metal reacts rapidly with exposed emulsion and influences the lighter shades (low contrast), thereby giving fine detail.

Activator

Developer is basically an alkaline and its alkalinity should be maintained throughout the development. Activator is used to maintain its alkalinity and chemical used is called alkali. The *alkali* adjusts the hydrogen ion concentration (pH), which affects the developing power of the developing agents. Activator also softens the gelatin, opens the pores of the film, and allows the developing agents to do their work. The alkali also serves as a buffer to control hydrogen ions liberated during development. Thus, activator enhances the action of the developer.

The most frequently used alkalies are *sodium hydroxide, sodium carbonate, potassium hydroxide, potassium carbonate,* and *sodium metaborate,* which swell gelatin, produce alkalinity and control the pH. The potassium salts have better advantage than sodium, since it has higher solubility. Sodium carbonate has been used as activator for many years. It causes gas formation in the emulsion, when the film is immersed in a cooler fixer. This leads to film blistering. To overcome this, the temperature of the developer, rinser, and the fixer solution should be the same. Sodium metaborate can be used at higher temperatures. It does not cause gas formation in the emulsion. It is the most efficient activator available today. The optimum pH of the activator ranges from 10 to 11.

Preservative

Developing agents absorb oxygen from air and easily get oxidized. Preservative is used to overcome the above issue. *Sodium sulfite* or *potassium sulfite* are used as preservatives. The preservative decreases the rate of oxidation of the hydroquinone, thereby increasing the life of the developer solution. Hydroquinone is more sensitive for aerial oxidation. Preservative helps to maintain proper development rate and also maintains balance among the developer components. The oxidation products of the developing agents decompose the alkaline solution and form colored materials that can stain the emulsion. The preservative dissolves these oxidation products and forms colorless sulfonates.

Restrainer

An ideal developing agent should react only with exposed silver bromide ions, rather than with unexposed AgBr ions. Restrainer is used to achieve the above purpose. Thus, the restrainer restricts the action of the developing agents only to those exposed AgBr crystals. *Potassium bromide* is used as restrainer, which is an *antifog agent*. It decreases the rate of fog formation, by protecting the unexposed crystals. Fog is the development of unexposed silver halide grains that do not contain the latent image. It also decreases the rate of development of the latent image, to a lesser degree. Thus, the restrainer improves the radiographic contrast, by reducing the fog. Potassium bromide can be used with *benzotriazole,* which can act at lower concentration.

Solvent

The solvent dissolves the chemicals and also helps for their ionization. It also aids in softening the gelatin emulsion. The commonly used solvent is water, which is freely available and cheap. The water should be soft water, if it is hard, the salts in the water will react with chemicals,

resulting in precipitates. In that case, water softener (*Calgon*) is added in the developer solution. Development depends on the following parameters:
◯ Crystal size
◯ Developer concentration
◯ Time
◯ Temperature.

Manufacturer's recommended concentration, time, and temperature must be employed to get optimal contrast, speed, and fog, otherwise it will reduce image quality. The usual developing time is 4–5 minutes for ordinary X-ray developer and 3 minutes for rapid X-ray developer at 68°F.

Rinsing

When the X-ray film is removed from the developer, it is saturated with all soluble chemicals contained in the developer. These chemicals include unoxidized developing agents and various oxidation products. Apart from these chemicals, the gelatin contains the black metallic silver and unexposed, undeveloped AgBr crystals. Hence, the developed film should be rinsed, in order to remove the soluble chemicals and oxidation products. Rinsing is done usually with water or acid.

Rinsing also partially stops the reaction of the developer and neutralizes the alkalinity of the residual developer. Thus, it reduces fog formation. If proper rinsing is not done, the developer may go to the fixer solution, resulting in *dichromic fog* and *brown staining* of the film. It increases the alkalinity of the fixer solution. Insufficient rinsing shortens the fixer life and also destroys its hardening action. Hence, stains may appear on the film.

In the water bath rinsing, the film is thoroughly rinsed in circulating water for 30 seconds. On removal from the rinse bath, it is placed in the fixing solution. Insufficient rinsing will disturb the chemical balance of the fixer and shorten the fixer life. Poor rinsing also reduces the acidity of the fixer and destroys its hardening action. Hence, stains may appear on the film. An acid rinse bath can be prepared by adding 2 liters of 28% acetic acid to 1 gallon of water. After thoroughly stirring, water is added to make 5 gallons (1 gallon = 4.55 liters) of solution. The film is rinsed for 30 seconds. The acid rinse bath is used to prolong the life of the fixer. It also maintains the hardening action of the fixer.

A combination of water and acid rinse bath procedure is the most efficient. In this method, the film is thoroughly rinsed for 5–10 seconds in running water. Later, it is placed in acid rinse bath for 15–30 seconds. It is then removed and placed in the fixer. Rinsing is not necessary for automatic film processor, where the transport rollers squeeze the film and wipe out residual developer.

Fixing

Fixing is the process of making the image permanent without fading. It is the removal of unexposed silver halides without damaging the image, formed by metallic silver. It also hardens the gelatin emulsion and stops residual development. The solution used for fixation is known as a fixing solution or *fixer*. The factors that influence the fixer are as follows:
- Type of fixer
- Concentration of the fixer
- Temperature of the solution
- Presence of hardeners
- Type of film material
- Agitation of the film
- Exhaustion of the fixing bath.

The fixing solution consists of the following composition:
- Solvent
- Activator
- Fixing agent
- Hardener
- Preservative
- Buffer
- Sequestering agent.

Solvent

The solvent is used to mix the chemical; usually *water* is used as solvent.

Activator

Sulfuric or *acetic acid* is used as acidifier. It neutralizes the alkalinity of the residual developer, still remaining on the film. It also provides a suitable medium for the fixer and hardener to act, thereby preventing the formation of stains.

Fixing Agent

The function of the fixing agent is to change the residual, unexposed, undeveloped AgBr crystals into soluble salts, without damaging the silver image. *Sodium* or *ammonium thiosulfate salts (hypo)* are used as common fixing agents. It dissolves the unexposed, undeveloped silver halides, leaving the developed metallic silver in the exposed areas of the film. The silver bromide reacts with sodium thiosulfate and form sodium bromide + sodium salt of *mono argento-di-thiosulphuric acid*. Similarly, the ammonium thiosulfate reaction can produce ammonium bromide + ammonium salt of *mono argento-di-thiosulphuric acid*. The later combination is less stable, but highly soluble in water and quickly washable.

Excess hypo, known as *hypo retention*, may cause oxidation and make image discolor, to brown, over a period of time. If the film is not fixed, the unexposed and undeveloped AgBr makes the radiograph nearly opaque and black. Silver combines with hypo and forms silver sulfide, which appears yellowish brown.

Hardener

The film coming out of the developer may absorb moisture and get swelled; hence, there is a need for hardening the emulsion. *Potassium alum, chromium alum,* and *aluminum chloride* are used as hardener. It hardens the gelatin emulsion, thereby protecting it from physical injuries. When the undeveloped silver bromide is removed from the film, the emulsion starts shrinking. The hardener enhances the shrinking process and makes the emulsion too hard. Now it is suitable for transport through washing and drying.

The pH of the hardener is very important. Higher pH may reduce the hardening efficiency. The recommended pH ranges of the hardeners are; potassium alum 4.5–4.9, chromium alum 3.5–4.7, and aluminum chloride 4.1–4.4, respectively. The following are the advantages of hardener:
- Drying is quicker, since gelatin absorbs less water
- Radiograph is less susceptible to external injury
- Driers can be operated at higher temperature.

Preservative

The pH of the fixer solution should be maintained as 4.0–5.0. To do this, *sodium sulfite* is used as preservative along with buffer, which maintains the chemical balance. The developer may mix with fixer solution and may cause chemical imbalance. Thus, preservative protects the fixing agent, from decomposition. It also helps in clearing the film and prevents residual developer. *Sodium acetate* is used as buffer, which keeps the pH of the fixer as constant. *Boric acid* and *boric salts* are used as sequestering agent, which removes metallic ions such as aluminum impurities. Insufficiently rinsed films may result in dichromic fog, streaks, and brown staining. This can be avoided, by adding a weak acid and a stabilizer in the fixer solution, e.g. *sodium metabisulfite* or *potassium metabisulfite*.

The fixing time depends on the age of the fixer and the number of films processed. A normal fixer takes about 1–4 minutes to clear the chemicals and 2–3 times the clearing time to harden the emulsion. A fixer is said to be exhausted, if the fixing time is >10 minutes. The film should not be exposed to white light during fixing. The optimum temperature for fixing bath is about 18–24°C.

Washing

After fixing, the film must be washed with water. This is to remove the residual processing chemicals and fixing-bath chemicals, especially hypo. If these chemicals are not removed, the image will discolor and fade, i.e.

the black silver will change into brown silver sulfide, resulting in *yellow brown stain*. Incomplete washing, permits the hypo retention, which may cause image fading, and make the film brown with age. Silver sulfite and other salts from the fixer deposit on the film surface, make it difficult to view the radiograph.

Normally, X-ray films should be washed in running water and it takes about 20 minutes. When the film is immersed in the water the thiosulfate from the film is removed by the water, by diffusion process. After some time, the diffusion stops, since the water has equal amount of thiosulfate. Therefore, the water should be replaced, that is why running water is preferred. The rate at which the thiosulfate is removed from film is known as *washing rate*. The washing rate depends upon the following factors:

- The type of X-ray film
- The rate at which water flows through the tank
- The temperature of water
- Type of fixing bath used and agitation of water.

Normally, washing takes about 20 minutes with running water at 20°C. The temperature of the water must be maintained at 25–30°C in automatic processor. There are two methods of washing, namely:

- Single tank washing
- Two-stage cascade system of washing.

In the single tank washing, the film should initially be placed near the outlet. After partial washing the film should be moved nearer the inlet, so that final washing is done in fresh uncontaminated water. The two-stage cascade system of washing is the efficient method. In this system, water flows in a direction opposite to the flow of films. The film is placed initially in the first compartment, where 90% of the salts are removed from the film. Later, the film is placed in the second compartment for fresh uncontaminated water washing.

When the water flow is 8 gallons per hour, the washing in each compartment takes only 5 minutes. In a manual processor multiple films are washed simultaneously, may take a time duration of 10 minutes. In an automatic processor 1–2 films are only washed at a time, and the time duration is about 18–20 seconds.

Drying

The final step in processing is to dry the radiograph. During the drying process, the radiographs are wet and easy to damage. The film may be dried in a dust free open air area, where the temperature is less than 35°C. Hence, films should not be removed from the hangers, until the drying is over. The speed with which the X-ray film dries, depends upon the quantity of water to be evaporated from the emulsion. To speed-up the drying process several drying aids are used. The most commonly used

X-ray Film Processing

wetting agent is *photo-flo* or *alcohol*. Photo-flo is used after final wash, to minimize water marks or streaks during development. It reduces the surface tension of the water, so that water can drain rapidly from the film surface.

Alcohol may be used for drying at emergency. After washing, the film is immersed in a tray of alcohol for 2 minutes at 70°F. Alcohol replaces water from the pores of the emulsion. The film is then drained. Most of the installations are provided with hot air drying cabinets. This is equipped with a fan and heating element to flow hot air. To flow air ordinary electric fan can also be used. The drying temperature must not exceed 35°C and the film must be hanged in a dust free area. In automatic processor warm dry air is blown over both surfaces of the film, while it is moving in the drying cabinet.

PREPARATION OF THE BATHS

The baths can be prepared either directly in the tank or in a pail. A pail is a cylindrical vessel made up of wood or tin or plastic, and having a handle with lid. If chemicals in powder form are used, then it is best to dissolve them in a pail, which should be a plastic or stainless steel. If concentrated solution is used for preparing the baths, then it can be diluted directly in the tank.

Developer Bath

Usually, the processing chemicals are provided as dry powders or as liquid solutions. A proper volume should be made by adding water as per the instruction. The commercially available developer powder is as pocket A and B. The pocket A is small, and the pocket B is big. The developer should be mixed carefully, as both chemicals (A and B) can cause burns. Suitable protecting clothing should be worn in the form of gloves, aprons, etc. One should also follow carefully the manufacturer's instructions. Let us take 6.75 liters of water in the developer tank and the pocket A is opened, and the chemical is poured slowly, by continuous stirring. Later the pocket B is opened and is poured and the stirring continues. Next sufficient water is added to make up to 13.5 liters working solution. The chemicals are stirred continuously at least for 2 minutes to give uniform mixture. Stirring is very important, as it prevents the formation of insoluble precipitates. Dissolving can be speeded up by increasing the water temperature (40°C/105°F).

Fixer Bath

The fixer powder is available in single pocket. Let us take 13.5 liters of warm water in the fixer tank. The pocket is opened and the chemical is poured slowly, by continuous stirring. Stirring is continued at least for 2 minutes to ensure a uniform mixture. Stirring is very vital to prevent

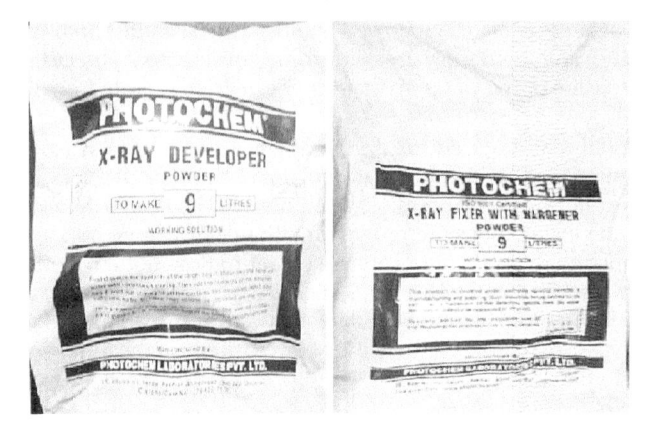

Fig. 5.2: Developer and fixer (Powder) for manual X-ray film processing. (*Courtesy*: M/s Photochem Laboratories Pvt. Ltd.)

localized production of insoluble sulfur particles. Separate stirring rods for developer and fixer, is very much essential. The fixer temperature is closely related to developer temperature. It should not be lesser than 2°C cooler than the developer. The commercial developer and fixer powder form are shown in Figure 5.2.

INFLUENCE OF TIME AND TEMPERATURE

Development is a chemical process, which depends on both temperature and time. Both temperature and time influence the developing. The time of development given to a film affects the amount of silver deposits. As the time of development increases, silver deposit also increases. As time decreases silver deposit also decreases. The time of development has a direct relation to the activity of the developer. In general, the time required to develop a film in a given developer depends upon the emulsion and thickness of film. There are two basic times of development, namely:
- Average speed of contrast
- Maximum speed of contrast.

The average speed contrast needs 25% more X-ray exposure, short time of development (4–5 minutes for ordinary X-ray developer and 3 minutes for rapid X-ray developer at 68°F). The maximum speed of contrast requires less than 25% X-ray exposure, longer time of development (6 minutes for ordinary X-ray developer and 5 minutes for rapid X-ray developer at 68°F).

The temperature change affects the chemical reactions. Variations in temperature require adjustment in the development time. Therefore, a good *thermometer* is essential to determine the correct temperature of the developer solution. The optimum temperature as recommended by the **American Standards Association** for developer is 20–22°C.

Higher temperature increases reduction of silver and enhances the number of silver grains. It is vice versa at lower temperature. At higher temperature, such as >24°C the emulsion becomes very soft and produces chemical fog. To overcome this, development time must be decreased. *One quarter (¼) of development time is decreased for 1° temperature increase.* A raise of 10° in temperature doubles the speed of the chemical reaction.

Films may be underdeveloped in low temperatures. Hence, the exposure time must be increased. At low temperature, such as <16°C the action of hydroquinone ceases and the resulting radiograph lacks contrast and density. This can be overcome by increasing the developer time. To achieve good development, *one-fourth minute of development is increased for 1° of temperature decrease*. In manual development, radiographic exposure is based on 5 minute development at 29°C, whereas it is 22 seconds in automatic processor. This will produce a radiograph of superior contrast with about 5 kV less exposure than is required for 3 minutes development. Processing of films on the above basis is called *time-temperature development.*

The other method of development is the *inspection method*. In this method, the film is often removed from the developer for inspection. This may result in slight fogging by oxidation in air. Hence, the inspection method is used only at emergency.

REPLENISHER

When the film is moved from the developing tank to rinsing bath, some quantity of developer accompanies the film and leads to loss of developer. This loss has to be replenished. Replenisher is used to restore the concentration of developer chemical to the original value. It also compensates the reduction in alkalinity and overcomes the accumulation of bromide. Normal replenisher contains a higher concentration of *hydroquinone, metal,* and *alkali*. Therefore, the chemicals are only exhausted, due to continuous development. The replenisher does not contain bromide, since it is released from the film emulsion.

With replenisher system, films should be removed quickly from the developer. One gallon (4.5 liters) of replenisher should be added for every 40 numbers of 14" × 17" films or their equivalent area. In properly replenished developer, one can develop 125 number of 14"× 17" films per gallon of solution. The solution should be discarded when the volume of replenisher used equals to three or four times the original quantity of the developer. The solution should also be discarded at the end of 3 months period though it is not used. Replenisher should never be added to the developer, while the films are developing. If it is added streaks of high density will be produced.

AUTOMATIC FILM PROCESSOR

Instead of manual processing, film processing is done automatically, which provides consistent and uniform quality radiographs. It was first introduced by **Pako** in 1942. In automatic processing, there are three important stages namely, *unloading the film, inserting into processor, and reloading the cassette,* whereas this is done in nine steps in manual processing. Hence, opportunities are there in manual processing for damage to the film or screens. An automatic processor runs the film sequentially through the developing, fixing, and washing solutions. The automatic processor consists of a number of separate, but interrelated systems listed below:
- Transport system
- Temperature control system
- Circulation system
- Replenishment system
- Drying system (Fig. 5.3).

Transport System

The transport system consists of the following parts:
- Feed tray
- Entrance rollers
- Microswitch
- Roller assembly
- Transport racks
- Drive motor.

The film is inserted into the feed tray at the darkroom. The shorter dimension of the film should always be against the side rail to maintain proper replenishment rate. The film should be fed evenly using the side rails of the feed tray. The entrance roller holds the film and begins its journey through the processor. A microswitch controls the replenishment rate of the chemicals. Later, the film is transported by rollers and racks through the developer and fixer solutions.

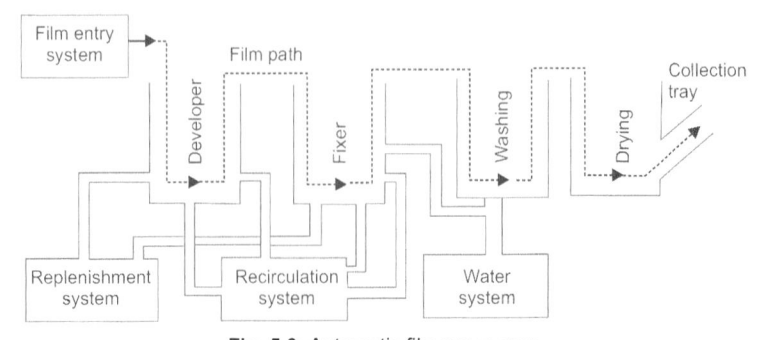

Fig. 5.3: Automatic film processor.

The transport system also controls the time during which the film is in the wet solution. For this purpose the transport system has the following:
○ Rollers
○ Transport racks
○ Drive motor.

Roller assembly consists of the following parts:
○ Transport rollers
○ Master roller
○ Planetary roller.

There are two types of rollers, namely:
○ Hard rollers
○ Soft rollers.

The transport rollers (1 in dia.) are in pairs, opposite to one another and keep the film in correct path. The master roller (3 in dia.) helps the film to turn around with the help of planetary rollers and guide shoes.

A crossover rack helps the film to move from one tank to another. It is made up of rollers and guide shoes. The racks contain stainless steel or plastic guide plates, which keep the film within the transport path. These guide plates must be kept clean, otherwise scratches may occur on the film. A drive motor of 10–20 rpm transfers power to the transport rack and drive the rollers, through a belt and pulley or chain and sprocket or gears. A shallow tank system is simple, cheaper, whereas deep rack system is costly, and is of high capacity.

Film Entry System

Every processor must have some apparatus, which will take the film into the processor (Fig. 5.4). Usually, this is linked to the replenishment system, so that the film entry activates the replenishment pumps for a period of time. An ideal film entry system consists of a pair of rollers and a microswitch above the rollers. There are many versions of microswitch, e.g. infrared light, stream of air, etc. which are interrupted by the film's entry. In the processor the lower roller is fixed and the top roller is made heavy with small movement. When the film is fed, the top roller moves upward and correspondingly the microswitch activates number of electrical systems. A warning in the form of bell or buzzer is used to tell when the next film is to be inserted.

Temperature Control System

Temperature of the developer, fixer, and water should be maintained precisely. The developer and wash water should be maintained at 35°C and 32°C, respectively. Hence, a heating element controlled by a thermocouple is provided for each tank. It controls the temperature of each solution.

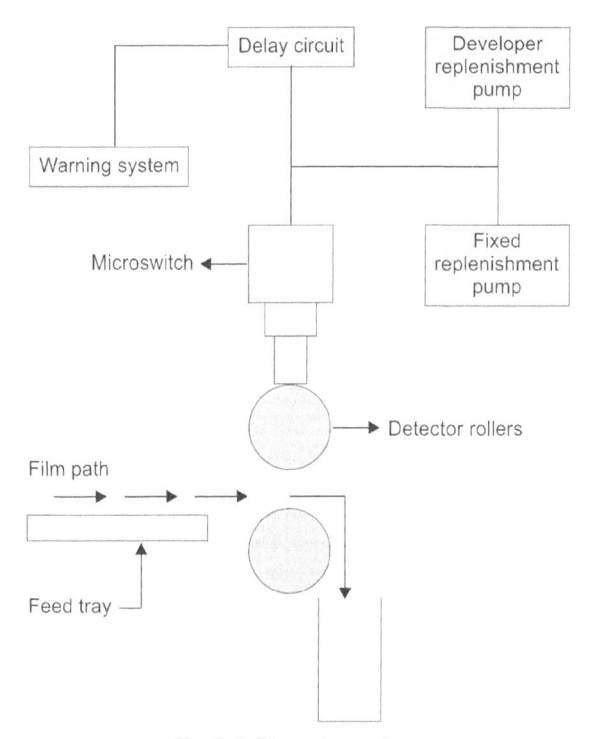

Fig. 5.4: Film entry system.

Circulation System

The circulation system consists of tanks for the following:
○ Developing
○ Fixing
○ Washing
○ Subsystems.

These tanks are made up of inert material such as *stainless steel* or *plastic*. This system is closely interrelated to the replenishment, water, and heating system. The chemicals in the tank must be circulated constantly and maintained at correct temperature. The developer and fixer solutions are constantly passed through the *thermostat, temperature gauze, heat exchanger, circulation pump, heater, and filter*. The thermostat controls the temperature, whereas thermometer measures the temperature. The heat exchanger is a part of the water system. Circulation pump is used to circulate developer through various devices. The filter helps to keep the developer clean.

The developer and fixer chemicals should be mixed by agitation, to have constant temperature. The circulation system pumps the chemicals

X-ray Film Processing

continuously, and provides agitation in each tank. In the developer, the circulation system filter the particles of 100 μm size released by the emulsion. Hence, these particles will not reach the rollers, thereby reducing artifacts. However, this is not 100% foolproof, *sludge* can build over a period of time. Such a filter system is not required in fixer tank; the fixer hardens and shrinks the gelatin. Further, fixer neutralizes the developer, the above said issue may not affect the final image.

Water is circulated in the wash tank in an open system, to remove all processing chemicals from the film. Usually, the inlet is provided at the bottom and the outlet is at the top, the water that overflows is fed into the sewage. The water overflows and comes out from the tank at the rate of 12 L/min.

Replenishment System

The replenishment system preserves both the quality and quantity of the chemicals in the processor. In every film processing, some amount of developer and fixer is absorbed. As a result, the chemical level in the tank drops and decreases the processing time. The replenishment system monitors this loss and preserves both quality and quantity of the chemicals in the processor, both in developer and fixer. It consists of the following:
- Replenisher tanks
- Filters
- Replenishment pumps.

These tanks are made up of stainless steel or plastic. But the developer replenisher tank has a floating lid to reduce auto-oxidation of developer replenisher solution.

When the film is inserted in the tray, a microswitch is activated, which switches ON the replenishment to a duration equal to film processing. This system helps the developer to maintain its *alkalinity and strength*. It also helps the fixer solution to maintain its *acidity and strength*. The replenishment rate is adjusted for each film processing. It is 60–70 mL for developer and 100–110 mL for fixer, for every 14 inches film. Developer replenisher is normally used for 2 weeks. Filters are made with stainless steel mesh, to prevent large particles, which may block the pump. The replenisher pump operates an electric motor, which fills the solutions up to tank level.

Water System

The water system is either cold water or tempered water system. This consists of the following:
- Cold and hot water supply
- Filters
- Mixing value
- Flow gauze
- Temperature gauze
- Heat exchanger.

The value controls the filtered water flow and temperature accurately. When the valve is set for a given temperature, it will maintain a constant flow of water. The flow gauge indicates the flow rate of water into the processor. The temperature gauge shows the operating temperature of the water. The heat exchanger box contains series of tubes through which water and developer is flowing. It absorbs waste heat from the developer and controls the developer temperature. In fixer, the heat exchanger passes the waste heat to the water from which it is reabsorbed by the fixer.

Dryer System

After processing, the radiograph is wet it may pickup dust, resulting in artifacts. Wet film is difficult to handle and viewing. Hence, there is a need of proper drying of the film. The dryer system consists of the following:
- Roller transport
- Blower
- Heater
- Ventilation ducts
- Drying tubes
- Air knives
- An exhaust system.

The roller transport system ensures that the speed of the film is same throughout the processor. The blower unit generates the airflow, which is blown over the heater. This system works on negative air pressure and absorbs moisture from the film. The blower sucks the room air and blow on the heating coils (2,500 W). Hence, room must be free of dust with low humidity. The temperature of the air entering system is monitored by a thermocouple. The drying tubes are positioned on both sides of the film and the hot moist air is vented out.

The temperature of the drying air is controlled by the *thermostat* and is usually about 50°C. The *air knives* are used to increase the velocity of the air, when it strikes the film surface. The combination of water and chemicals with electricity could be fatal. To avoid this, great care must be taken in the installation of an automatic processor. Various standards are specified in different countries in order to maintain electrical safety and pollution effects, etc. There is also a need for standby system, which automatically shuts down, if the film has not entered the processor within the given time. A typical interval is of 2 minutes for a 90 seconds automatic film processor. The standby system will reduce the running cost reasonably.

Advantage of Automatic Film Processor

The automatic processor is very much suitable to a busy X-ray department. It reduces the processing time (90 s), and improves the efficiency, workflow, and image quality. The advantages of automatic processor are as follows:

X-ray Film Processing

- Time in the developer, fixer, washer and dryer is constant, due to controlled drive system.
- The temperature of all the solution is unaffected by outside environmental conditions.
- The quality and quantity of the solutions are maintained to a high standard, due to automatic replenishment.
- Due to circulation, uniform penetration of the chemicals into the emulsion layer of the film is achieved by constant agitation.
- Even drying and uniform surface quality of the film is obtained, due to constant dryer temperature.
- Satisfactory results can be obtained even with exposure discrepancies as great as ±25%.
- Total processing time is less.

SOLUTIONS FOR AUTOMATIC PROCESSOR

Developer

Automatic processing solutions have special features that make them quite different from manual processing solutions. In the case of automatic processor, reference will be made as developer replenisher and machine tank developer, i.e. developer replenisher + starter solution = machine tank developer. The probable developer constituents are as follows:

- Developing agents
- Preservative
- Accelerator
- Restrainer (antifoggant)
- Buffer
- Sequestering agent
- Solvent
- Other additions such as hardening agent, wetting agent antifoggant, fungicide, etc.

The majority of the chemical's name and function are similar to that of manual processing. *Boric acid + sodium hydroxide* is used as *buffer*. Its main function is to maintain the pH within defined limits and thereby maintains the activity of the developer constant. *The ethylene diamine tetra-acetic acid (EDTA) sodium salt* is used as sequestering agent. Its main function is to soften the hard water. The hardening agent reduces swelling and softening. The wetting agent reduces surface tension. The antifoggant prevents foaming due to reduced surface tension. The fungicide reduces growth of fungi.

The commercial preparations are available in liquid concentrate, packed in three parts namely, A, B, and C (Fig. 5.5). Each of the three parts comprises various items as follows:

Part A: Developing agent (*hydroquinone*), preservative (*sulphite*), buffer + accelerator

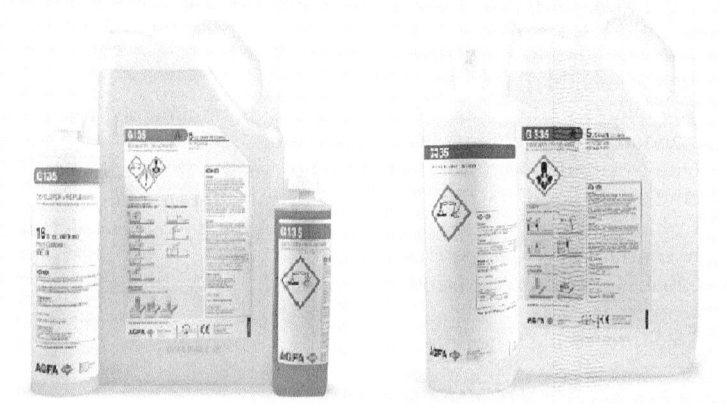

Fig. 5.5: Developer and fixer in liquid form for automatic X-ray film processing. (*Courtesy*: M/s Agfa Healthcare India Pvt. Ltd.)

Part B: Developing agent (*phenidone*),
   Solvent for phenidone (*diethylene glycol*)
   Restrainer (*Potassium bromide, acetic acid*)
Part C: Hardener (*Glutaraldehyde*)
   Acetic acid

The mixing of the chemicals is to be carried out as per the instructions given by the manufacturer. The method of mixing is as follows: Let us take the volume of water as stated in the instructions. Add slowly the whole parts of A, B, and C, with continuous stirring. Continue stirring for at least 2 minutes to give a uniform mixture.

Fixer

The fixing solution consists of the following composition:
- Fixing agent (*ammonium thiosulfate*)
- Acid (*acetic acid or sulfuric acid*)
- Buffer (acetic acid)
- Preservative (*sodium or potassium sulfite*)
- Hardener (*aluminum chloride + acetic acid*)
- Solvent (*water*).

The commercial preparations are available as liquid concentrate in two parts namely A and B as follows:
Part A: Fixing agent, acid, buffer, preservative, solvent
Part B: Hardener, acid.

The mixing of the chemicals is to be carried out as per the instructions given by the manufacturer. The method of mixing is as follows: Take the volume of water as stated in the instructions. Add slowly the whole part of A with continuous stirring. Add the whole part of B or the correct amount (25 mL per liter) according to the instructions. Continue stirring at least for 2 minutes to ensure a uniform mixture.

Difference between Manual and Automatic Film Processing

Apart from the above, automatic processing eliminates use of hangers, requires lesser water consumption, reduces film wastage, saves space, and helps in processing large number of films. The electrical consumption and chemical costs are almost same, both in manual and automatic processing. The processing time difference between the manual processing and automatic film processor is given in Table 5.1. The major differences between manual and automatic film processing is given in Table 5.2.

Silver Recovery

Used fixer solution contains silver. Hence, it should not be disposed directly to the drainage or sewage. It has to be collected in container for silver recovery. It may contain about 1 g silver per liter. The reasons for silver recovery are as follows:
○ It is a declining natural source
○ Fixer effluent can cause ecological damage
○ Higher price.

The various methods of silver recovery are follows:
○ Metal (ion) exchange
○ Electrolytic recovery
○ Chemical method
○ Galvanic method.

In the metal (ion) exchange method base metals (steel wool or zinc) are used for extraction. When the fixer solution is in contact with the base metal, the silver replaces the base metal, and the base metal ions are released into the solution. The sludge containing the silver is dried and refined. The efficiency of this method is about 70%.

In the electrolytic method, two electrodes are used. *Carbon anode* and *stainless steel cathode* are placed in the fixer solution. A direct current

Table 5.1: Processing time difference between manual and automatic.		
Process	Manual	Automatic
Developing	3–5 min	22 s
Rinsing	10–20 s	Nil
Fixing	10 min	22 s
Washing	15 min	22 s
Drying	20 min	24 s
Total (approximately)	50 min	90 s

Table 5.2: Difference between manual and automatic film processing.

S. No.	Manual film processing	Automatic film processing
1.	There are 9 steps: ➢ Unloading the film ➢ Loading the film in hanger ➢ Development ➢ Rinsing ➢ Fixing ➢ Washing ➢ Wetting agent ➢ Drying ➢ Reloading the cassette	There are 3 steps: ➢ Unloading the film ➢ Feeding into the processor ➢ Reloading the cassette
2.	Require film hangers	No need of film hangers
3.	Water flow is continuous	Water flows only while the film is in the processor
4.	Cold water is used	Water temperature is maintained at 25–30°C
5.	Water consumption is high; 12–15 L/min	Water consumption is less; 1.5 L/min
6.	Film wastage is high	Film wastage is less
7.	One technician can process maximum of only 5 m^2/h films	Maximum processing may go up to 15 m^2/h films
8.	Overall space required is large	Require lesser space
9.	Day light processing is not possible	Day light processing is possible
10	Electrical and chemical costs are similar	Electrical and chemical costs are similar

is passed in between the electrodes. The silver ions (Ag$^+$) move toward the cathode, where it is neutralized and become metallic silver. It can be operated either as low current or high current density. The silver deposition is faster in the latter mode. This is the most efficient method, and can offer recovery of up to 95%.

In chemical method, certain chemicals are added to the fixer solution. The silver is separated in the form of precipitate. In the galvanic method, dissimilar metals in contact with other are immersed in the fixer. The silver is deposited in the metal plate, which can be collected.

Recovery of Silver from Used X-ray Films

Exposed X-ray films have certain amount of silver. It consists of about 4 g of silver per square meter of film. The amount of silver recovery depends on the amount of fixer used during a given period. There are agencies who can buy the films by weight (kg) and extract silver by any one of the above method.

Processor Quality Assurance

Quality assurance (QA) is a tool by which one can evaluate the tolerance or the performance of an equipment/procedure. Film processing require QA protocol in assessment of film storage conditions, darkroom fog and cleanliness, processor chemistry analysis, replenishment and developer temperature measurements, and mechanical integrity of the processor. Since these parameters undergo changes from day-to-day, it is necessary that QA needs to be performed daily before taking clinical images. Logbook involving QA data is to be maintained, to predict trends and tolerance conditions. Whenever tolerance is exceeded, suitable corrective measures need to be undertaken.

Film is sensitive to pressure, heat, humidity, and chemical fumes. They should be stored in vertical (on edge). Room temperature and humidity (40–60%) must be maintained. Low humidity can cause static marks, by static electricity, whereas high humidity can cause stickiness in films, so that transport becomes difficult thereby causing fingerprint artifacts. Room must be kept clean and dust free; dust can mimic a variety of pathologies and make the film useless. The darkroom illumination must be optimum, so that fogging does not occur. Orthochromatic (green) films require red light, whereas blue sensitive films (calcium tungstate) are safe even in yellow light.

White light leaks can cause background fog on all films, particularly in mid-density regions, which contains important information. This will increase the film speed apparently, by decreasing film contrast. Hence, film fog test must be done once in 6 months. Processor chemistry analysis, developer temperature measurements and reproducibility of optical density levels are carried out on daily basis, before beginning the work.

To carry out the QA program the department requires a medical physicist. QA will take reasonable amount of time but save lot of money on chemical costs.

MULTIFORMAT IMAGING

Radiology departments prefer production of images in an electronic form, which has several advantages. Initially, the diagnostic monitor image was photographed by a *Polaroid camera* or a camera with radiographic film. With the advent of computed tomography (CT) scan and magnetic resonance imaging (MRI), there was a need to record more number of images in a single film. This is known as multiformat imaging. These images come in a variety of format, as many as 25 images on one film. There are mainly two systems, namely:
- Imaging camera
- Laser camera.

Imaging Camera

In the past, imaging cameras were linked to the monitor (bolt on type). A double-sided, dark slide cassette was provided. The film is loaded into both sides of the cassette. When the slide is removed, the film gets exposed. Then the film is covered with the slide and the procedure is repeated for the second film. Later cameras used flat screen monitor which accept only one size film, with specific format. For example, a 10" × 8" film will print only 0–4 images.

Later multiformat cameras are provided with microprocessor control and an inbuilt processing machine. They allow a single 17" × 14" film to record images from different format sizes. This system has a *flat faced monitor cathode-ray tube* (CRT), to avoid edge distortion (Fig. 5.6). The video output is recorded on the film with desired format. Then the film is passed onto the processor and after the completion of processing, the hard copy comes out. If there is no inbuilt processing, then the film goes to the magazine, from which it can be taken to the processing system. The camera efficacy is mainly controlled by the type of monitor, stability, exposure, interlacing, and lens system. One can use either paper or film to record the hard copy. The film has high spatial and temporal resolution over paper image, whereas paper images require no processing chemicals, but cost per image is high. These cameras are available for darkroom processing as well as daylight processing. Individual user should select what kind of system is needed for their use.

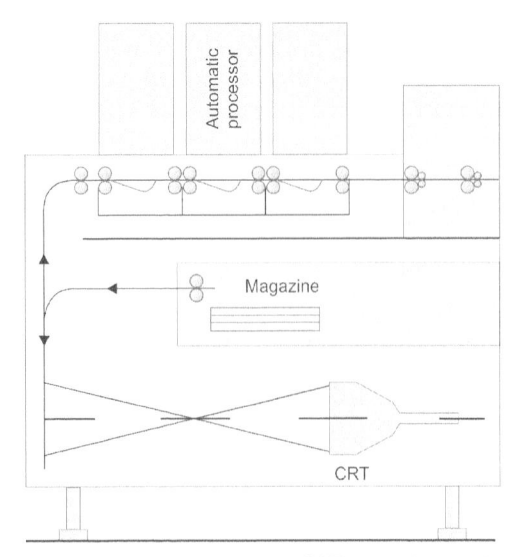

Fig. 5.6: The imaging camera. (CRT: cathode-ray tube)

X-ray Film Processing

This system needs a special film which has single side emulsion, with peak sensitivity of 540 nm. CT/MRI image has a black background and hence, the monitor image background is white, whereas ultrasound image has white background, hence, the monitor background is black. Because of this, CT/MRI requires a high contrast film, whereas ultrasound requires a low contrast film.

Laser Camera

Laser is abbreviated for light amplification by stimulated emission of radiation. Laser produces coherent beams of parallel light. Laser imager is an optical, electronic and mechanical device, which produces hard copy by exposing a film to laser light. It uses a *helium-neon laser* with emission of red light (632 nm). It contains a number of separate modules, namely:

- The laser
- An interference
- Memory store
- An acoustic-optical modulator
- An optical system
- Scanner
- Film transport system (Fig. 5.7).

In this, all the digital image information required for one film is stored in the memory, through the interference. The stored information is used to modulate the laser beam via an acoustic-optical modulator, in terms of brightness and gray levels, etc. The intensity of the beam is controlled by digital value of the input signal. A lens system is used to focus the laser beam onto a mirror, which moves the laser beam from side-to-side across the film. At a time one line of information is printed, which will contain 3,500–4,100 pixels. After each line is printed, the film moves vertically to allow the next line. The printing process takes about 8–30 seconds. Then the film is fed into the automatic processing unit.

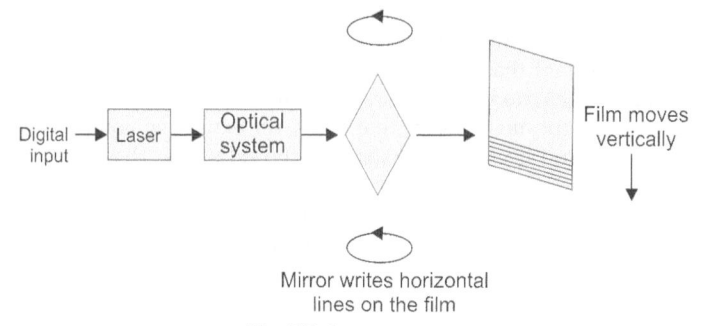

Fig. 5.7: Laser camera.

Laser camera requires single-sided, fine grain polyester-based silver halide film. Correct films should be purchased to match the type of laser. Helium-neon laser requires film which has sensitivity at 632 nm. *Green safe light filters* are required for darkroom handling.

Both imaging camera and laser camera have identical resolution. Data transfer time is short in the former. The magnetic field in MRI may affect imaging camera images, hence, proper care is needed in shielding the camera. Laser images are susceptible to dust and vibration, thereby producing artifacts on the image. Overall, laser images are superior, when used as a large format single image, where the image is produced from a high-resolution matrix, whereas imaging cameras are suitable for general imaging, where resolution matrix and format size is lower.

CHEMICAL POLLUTION

The degree of pollution caused by X-ray film processing is low, compared to other industries. However, appropriate steps should be taken to reduce chemical pollution to acceptable levels. This will preserve the environment for future generations.

The temperature of the liquid waste from X-ray processing does not exceed 37°C. The waste water should neither create obnoxious smells nor have discoloration. The dissolved solids present in the waste include *chlorides, sulfates, phosphates, leads, aluminum*, etc. In addition, the waste also consists of poisonous materials which will kill living organisms in the water. There is also a nutrient, which is not poisonous, but can upset the ecological balance by promoting the uncontrolled growth of plants and algae. Hence, the effluent discharge from the processor is diluted many times.

Many metallic ions have a serious effect on microorganisms and fish. Ideally, none of these should be discharged into any sewerage system. Silver is the most used in the X-ray processing. It is usually found as *thiosulfate* compound in the wash water. This is less toxic than pure silver. In addition, any silver ion present will form insoluble salts when combined with chloride, bromide, and sulfide ions.

It is important that the effluent from any silver recovery unit is to be checked, so that no silver is being discharged from the unit. The head of the department must ensure that the silver extracting company/firm is responsible and licensed to dispose of the solutions. These steps can reduce the environmental effect of the discharges of waste solutions.

Hence, a regular quality assurance program can be adopted, so that pollution can be reduced to an absolute minimum.

6
Screen-film Image Quality, Artifacts and Quality Assurance

IMAGE QUALITY

Radiographic image quality refers the visibility of a given anatomy as well as the accuracy of its structural lines recorded. A good radiograph should represent the anatomy accurately and it should be visualized well for further interpretation. The radiographic image quality can be divided into *visibility* and *image sharpness*. Visibility refers brightness and contrast of the image. Structural accuracy/image sharpness depends on special resolution, noise, distortion and the influence of geometric factors of the image. For a good quality image, the spatial resolution should be maximum and distortion should be minimum. To describe visibility of a radiography, the term image *clarity* (**R.E.Wayrymen**) was used. There is no standard way to describe image quality. However, it can be discussed in the following headings, as shown in the Figure 6.1A: The displayed factors are said to be primary factors, which can influence the image quality in a higher degree. There are also secondary factors, which can also affect the image quality in a lesser degree (Fig. 6.1B). However, the image quality mainly depends on;

○ Brightness
○ Contrast
○ Spatial resolution
○ Sharpness
○ Noise.

Brightness

Brightness is the amount of luminescence or light emission in the radiograph. *Density* is the degree of blackness of the image on the processed film. In general, a radiograph must have sufficient brightness

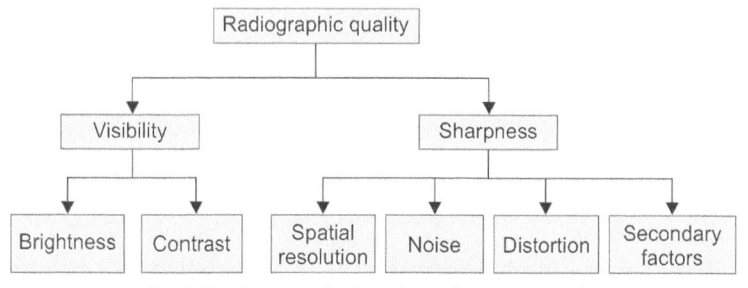

Fig. 6.1A: Factors affecting the radiographic quality.

Medical X-ray Film Processing

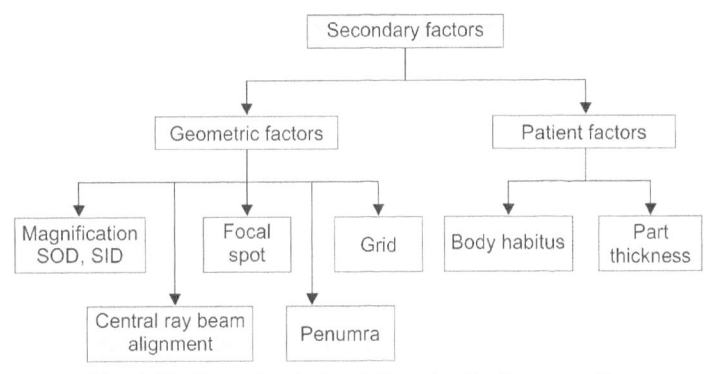

```
                        Secondary factors
                              │
              ┌───────────────┴───────────────┐
         Geometric factors               Patient factors
              │                               │
    ┌─────┬───┴──┬──────┐              ┌──────┴──────┐
Magnification Focal  Grid              Body habitus  Part
  SOD, SID    spot                                thickness
    │           │
Central ray  Penumra
beam alignment
```

Fig. 6.1B: Secondary factors influencing the image quality.

or density to see anatomical structures of interest. A radiograph of high brightness will have lesser density and difficult to view anatomical details. On the other hand, radiograph with little brightness will have excess density, and again limits the visualization of anatomy. What is needed is the optimal brightness and density. This depends upon the technical factors (kV, mA, S), which control the radiation reaching the film. In the case of screen-film radiography, the amount of radiation reaching the film has direct effect on density, whereas it has little impact in digital radiography.

Contrast

The term *contrast* refers the difference in density between adjacent areas in the radiograph. An image of insufficient density with no differences in density, appears as homogeneous object. This is due to the equal absorption characteristics of the object. If the absorption characteristics of the object differs, the image will have varying level of density, which is called *differential absorption*. Tissues that attenuate the X-ray beam equally are more difficult to visualize. It is easy to visualize images, in which tissue transmit X-rays unequally, so that there will be density difference, resulting in contrast. Hence, density difference generally refers radiographic contrast. It is mainly made up of by the following parameters:
- Subject contrast
- Film/image contrast (detector)
- Fog and scatter.

The product of subject contrast and film contrast gives the radiographic contrast.

Subject Contrast

Subject contrast is the difference in X-ray intensities transmitted through different parts of the patient, which depends on the following factors:

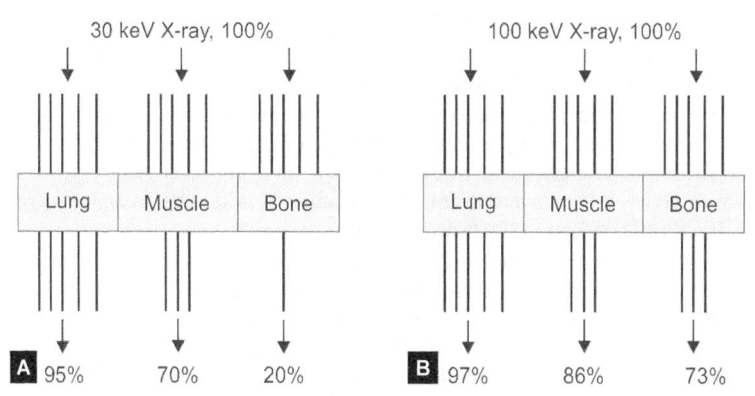

Screen-film Image Quality, Artifacts and Quality Assurance

```
30 keV X-ray, 100%              100 keV X-ray, 100%
   ↓    ↓    ↓                     ↓    ↓    ↓
 ┌────┬──────┬──────┐            ┌────┬──────┬──────┐
 │Lung│Muscle│ Bone │            │Lung│Muscle│ Bone │
 └────┴──────┴──────┘            └────┴──────┴──────┘
   ↓    ↓    ↓                     ↓    ↓    ↓
 A 95%  70%  20%                 B 97%  86%  73%
```

Figs. 6.2A and B: Effect of body anatomy and photon energy on X-ray beam intensity.

- Patient thickness
- Tissue mass density
- Effective atomic number
- Shape of the subject
- Photon energy (kVp).

Thicker and thinner body parts attenuate radiation differently, and vary the transmitted X-rays, leading to subject contrast. It can be positive, if the tissue absorbs fewer X-rays compared to the surroundings. Positive contrast always results in darker images, e.g. lung. On the other hand, negative contrast results in lighter image of the tissue. In the case of negative contrast, the tissue absorbs more X-rays than the surroundings, e.g. bone.

The subject contrast is proportional to the relative number of transmitted X-rays. Tissues of equal thickness, having different mass density contribute to subject contrast (Figs. 6.2A and B). Higher is the density of the tissue, greater the attenuation of the beam. From the figure, it is understood that bone absorbs 80% X-rays, whereas muscle absorbs 30% only, for 30 keV X-ray energy. The corresponding transmission is about 20% and 70%, respectively. As the X-ray energy increases to 100 keV, the transmission also increases to 73% and 86%, respectively for bone and muscle. However, the bone absorption remains high (27%), compared to muscle (14%). In the case of lung, the increase of X-ray energy has very little influence, due to its low mass density. The mass density of lung is 3 times lower than that of muscle. Photoelectric absorption varies with effective atomic number. If the adjacent tissue's effective atomic number is different, X-ray transmission varies and contribute subject contrast. Higher is the atomic number, greater the attenuation, due to photoelectric absorption.

Contrast media such as *Barium* ($Z = 56$), and *Iodine* ($Z = 53$) will enhance subject contrast. Barium has high density and atomic number, and offers high attenuation due to its K-edge of 37 keV. Similar is the case of iodine, that has the K-edge of 33 keV, matching the diagnostic energy range of X-rays. In addition, air (negative contrast agent) and *carbon dioxide* (angiography) are also used as contrast agents, that increase subject contrast. Chest is having bone, fat, and lung (air) tissues of varying X-ray transmission. Hence, chest radiograph will have more subject contrast, compared to abdomen and thorax. Hence, chest is said to be an anatomy of high natural contrast in the human body.

Shape of the anatomy, which coincides with the X-ray beam, increases the subject contrast. Shape that has change in thickness for X-ray path may reduce subject contrast. X-ray beam quality affects the subject contrast. High kVp gives lower subject contrast, whereas low kVp gives higher subject contrast. In high kV, the penetration power is increased, which decreases the attenuation, resulting in lesser absorption. At the same time it increases X-ray transmission and offers low subject contrast. High kV can be achieved by increasing the tube voltage, or adding filters or reducing ripple of the tube voltage. In the case of CT scan, increase of applied voltage reduces soft tissue contrast. At the same time, reduction of tube voltage improves the subject contrast with iodinated contrast agents.

Film Contrast

The film contrast or image contrast is the difference in film density of a lesion, compared to the film density of the adjacent tissues. Thus, the image contrast mainly depends on film density and film amplifies the subject contrast. The film contrast tells us how the film responds to difference in exposure. Underexposed films have low densities (0.5 OD), results in poor image contrast. Overexposed films (>2.0 OD) have high densities, and also result in poor image contrast. The desired density is 1.5 OD, which can provide optimal image contrast. This can be achieved by selecting correct image receptor or automatic exposure control. The film contrast depends on the following parameters:
○ Characteristic curve
○ Film density
○ Screen or non-screen exposure
○ Film processing.

Mainly, the slope (gradient) of the characteristic curve determines the film contrast. The recommended film gradient is about 2, whereas it is >3 for mammography. High gradient films are generally said to be high contrast films. High contrast film is made up of homogeneous size of silver grains, whereas low contrast film is made up of heterogeneous grains. Double emulsion films produce greater contrast than single emulsion films. The fog and scatter will reduce film contrast. They produce unwanted film density, which lowers final radiographic contrast. Film contrast has been discussed in detail in the earlier Chapter 3.

Film latitude is inversely proportional to film gradient. Low latitude films have higher film gradient, resulting in higher contrast. In these films, the range of air kerma values are narrow. These films are said to be high contrast films and use of high kV gives better subject contrast. Similarly, a wide latitude films have lower film gradient, resulting in low contrast. In these films, the range of air kerma values is wider. These films are said to be low contrast films and use of low kV will offer better subject contrast. In chest radiography, wide latitude films are often used, due to large difference between the air kerma values of lung and mediastinum. Mammography preferably uses low latitude films of higher contrast with breast compression.

Fog and Scatter

The fog and scatter will produce unwanted film density which lowers radiographic contrast. Generally, the term base + fog is used, which appear in the toe portion of the characteristic curve. Fog is the inherent blackness without any radiation exposure. Base refers the density of the film base. Improper storage of films may increase fog level, that reduces contrast. Accidental exposures of films to light also will increase fog level. Base + fog levels should not exceed greater than 0.2 OD. The following situations may increase the fog level:

- Improper film storage
- Developer solution (Both contaminated and exhausted)
- Higher darkroom temperature
- Long developing time
- Use of high speed films.

Scattered radiation arises due to Compton scattering. It increases with increase of the following factors:

- Patient thickness
- Field size
- Photon energy.

Scattered radiation that reaches the film may produce unwanted film density. Hence, subject contrast is reduced by the presence of scattered radiation. Scattered radiation is minimized by proper collimation. Use of grid to avoid scattered radiation will always improve subject contrast.

Overall, density is measurable, whereas contrast is a complex parameter to quantify. Evaluation of a radiograph in terms of contrast is more subjective. The optimal level of contrast required varies with nature of examination. The contrast required in chest radiograph is different from that of extremities.

However, the subject contrast is not only the factor to decide the overall image contrast. The combination of subject contrast and film contrast will decide the overall image contrast.

Resolution

Resolution is the ability to image two closely placed small objects, as two independent images. It is a measure of the radiograph's ability to differentiate between different structures that are close together. It tells about the screen-film combination's ability and how much detail that it can provide. There are three types of resolution namely:
- Spatial resolution
- Contrast resolution
- Temporal resolution.

Spatial resolution refers the ability of the imaging system to record the object in two special dimensions (x, y) of the image. In other words, it is the ability to image small objects that have high subject contrast, e.g. bone-soft tissue interface. Spatial resolution is often used with the terms like high contrast resolution, or sharpness or blur. If an image appear as sharp and distinct, then the system resolution is high. If the system resolution is low, then the image appears blurred. Spatial resolution is affected by the following factors:
- Focal spot size
- Detector blur
- Patient motion.

Contrast resolution is the ability to distinguish anatomical structures of similar subject contrast, e.g. liver-spleen. In general, screen-film radiography has excellent spatial resolution, whereas CT has superior contrast resolution. Temporal resolution is the ability of the imaging system to localize the object in time, from frame to frame and follow its movement. Temporal resolution is high for fluoroscopy.

Point Spread Function

To measure spatial resolution, number of functions are defined, as given below:
- Point-spread function (PSF)
- Line-spread function (LSF)
- Edge-spread function (ESF)
- Modulation transfer function (MTF).

The image produced for a single point object is called PSF, e.g. imaging a lead sheet that has tiny hole (10 μm) or performing CT scan on a wire, kept perpendicular to the slice plane. Then the image profile is measured by a densitometer, which gives the PSF (Fig. 6.3). The point appears blurred due to the effects of focal spot, motion and size of the detector. The dimension of the profile is measured at half width, which is called *full width half maximum (FWHM)*. If, the separation of two-point sources is greater than the FWHM, they can be resolved. The presence of scatter radiation will broaden the FWHM, with extended tails, which creates higher image blur or unsharpness.

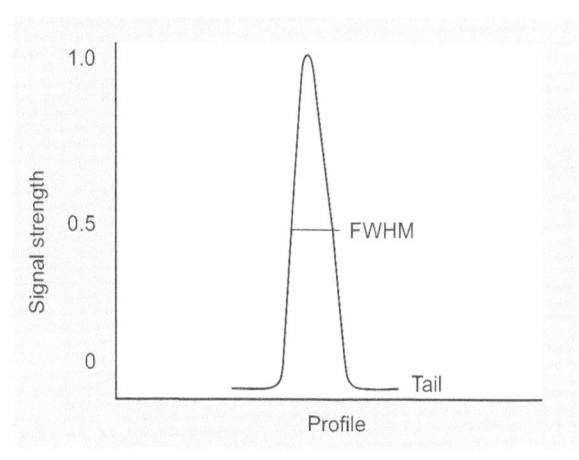

Screen-film Image Quality, Artifacts and Quality Assurance

Fig. 6.3: Point spread function.
(FWHM: Full width half maximum)

Line Spread Function

Though PSF describes the response of the imaging system, it represents a discrete point in the image surface and it is not suitable for system like screen-film, involving fixed area. Hence, functions like LSF and ESF are recommended. LSF describes the response of an imaging system to a linear stimulus. That is, it is an image of a narrow line source and its width (FWHM) is a measure of blur. In this, imaging is done with a slit (10 μm, platinum), and 90° image profile is measured, by a *densitometer*. This can be measured for both vertical and horizontal axis. Similarly, ESF is measured in fluoroscopy, using a sharp edge. A wide LSF refers poor spatial resolution, whereas narrow LSF refers good resolution. It is difficult to measure narrow LSF, <1 mm and *bar phantoms* are generally used to measure such spatial resolution. Bar patterns are made up of bars of lead and radiolucent material of equal width (0.5 mm), arranged in parallel. It has highest intrinsic contrast (Chapter 4). Wide LSFs are easy to measure with FWHM, e.g. nuclear medicine. The FWHM and spatial resolution (lp/mm) are related as follows:

$$FWHM = 1/(2 \times LSF)$$

For example, a spatial resolution of 1 lp/mm is equal to a FWHM of 0.5 mm.

The easiest way of describing the resolution is line pair (lp), in frequency domain. A line pair is a line of a particular width, followed by a space of the same width. It refers a bright stripe and an adjacent dark stripe in the image and its unit is lp/mm. This is in analogy to a sound wave (sine) having frequency in cycles/mm. Objects of an image that are

104 Medical X-ray Film Processing

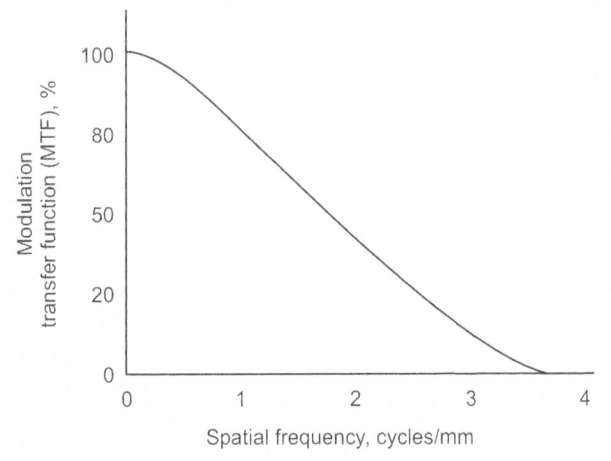

Fig. 6.4: Resolution capability of an imaging system.

separated by small distance (mm), possess high spatial frequency, similar to sound waves. If Δ is the size of the object, then spatial frequency (F) = 1/2Δ. For example, if object size is 0.5 mm, then spatial frequency is 1/(2 × 0.5) = 1 lp/mm. The human eye can resolve about 5 lp/mm at a viewing distance of 25 cm. In other words, in 5 lp/mm, there are 5 lines and 5 spaces within 1 mm and each line/space is of 0.10 mm width.

Modulation Transfer Function

Modulation transfer function (MTF) is the ratio of the recorded signal frequency (output contrast) to original signal frequency (input contrast) and it is always less than 1. That is, the output is always less than 100% due to blur offered by the focal spot, motion and detector size;

$$MTF = \frac{\text{Recorded signal}}{\text{Available signal}}$$

It is basically a curve, that describes the resolution capability of an imaging device. For an imaging system, it is plotted with spatial frequency versus MTF, for a given frequency (Fig. 6.4). Lower spatial frequency corresponds to bigger objects that have higher MTF, close to 1. Higher spatial frequency corresponds to smaller objects that have lower MTF values closer to zero. An imaging system usually consists of several components as in fluoroscopy, and hence, each component's MTF should be taken into account. The total MTF of a system is the product of all the component's individual MTF. It is calculated from the measurements of LSF.

Thus, MTF is useful to quantify the resolution of each component in an imaging system. In day-to-day practice, measurement of spatial resolution is done, by using star phantoms in radiography and line pair phantoms in computed tomography.

Screen-film Resolution

Film without screen has a spatial resolution of about 100 lp/mm, which depends on the silver grain size. Resolution is influenced by focal spot size, image sharpness (blur), and patient motion. The screen thickness used in radiology ranges from 50 μm to 400 μm. Thicker screens offer greater light diffusion and increases blur. Therefore, shorter exposure time is recommended to minimize screen blur. The resolution of screen-film radiography is 5–10 lp/mm, for 200 speed system. The required resolution in mammography is about 15 lp/mm. Accreditation agencies like American College of Radiology (ACR), recommend spatial resolution of about 11–13 lp/mm for screen-film radiography. That may be 13 lp/mm along the anode-cathode axis and 11 lp/mm perpendicular to the axis.

Image Sharpness

Image sharpness is the ability of the X-ray film or screen-film combination to define an edge. Due to light diffusion in the screen, the screen-film system may fail to record a sharp edges. This is known as image *unsharpness*. A system may have ability to record sharp images, but fail to resolve fine details. In contrast, images with unsharp edges may reveal fine details. Thus, sharpness and resolution are different, but interrelated. Unsharpness may be classified as follows:
○ Geometric unsharpness
○ Absorption unsharpness
○ Detector unsharpness
○ Motion unsharpness.

The geometric unsharpness arises from the focal spot size. The X-rays coming slightly different locations in the focal spot, produces blurred margin at the edge of the objects. This is called *penumbra*, which results in loss of sharpness, known as *focal spot blur*. Penumbra is a region at the beam edges, having variable intensity that decreases towards outside. The penumbra width increases with increase of focal spot size.

In contact radiography the focal spot blur is zero. This increases with increasing focal spot size and it is minimum in extremity radiography. Focal spot blur increases with magnification. Therefore, small focal spot size (0.1 mm) is always recommended for magnification radiography. Such a setup will not only reduce penumbra but also the image blur. It has the additional benefit of better visibility of micro-calcifications.

Absorption unsharpness arises, if the patient do not have objects that have sharp edges. This is due to gradual change of X-ray absorption towards the edges of an object. It produces a poorly defined margin in the image. This unsharpness increases for round and oval anatomy, e.g. coronary angiogram.

Detector blur is due to screens used in screen-film radiography. Screen unsharpness is caused by light diffusion in the intensifying screen. Thicker screens have greater light diffusion, whereas thin screens have lesser light diffusion. Thicker screen (>0.4 mm) produces lateral light diffusion, resulting in blurred images. The screen blur increases with separation of the film from the screen. Screen blur decreases with increase of resolution, crystal size, and contrast, but has limited value in assessing system performance.

Patient motion introduces unsharpness into the radiograph, which is called *motion blur*, e.g. heart motion. Movement of focal spot during the exposure can also cause motion artifacts. This can be minimized by increasing the mA, to reduce the exposure time. Shorter exposure always reduces motion unsharpness. Use of faster screen also decreases motion unsharpness. Immobilization devices and compression paddle (mammography) can be used, to reduce motion blur. There is no motion blur in magnification radiography. The total unsharpness (U_T) of an image is given as follows:

$$U_T = \sqrt{U_g^2 + U_a^2 + U_d^2 + U_m^2}$$

where, U_g^2 = geometric unsharprness
U_a^2 = absorption unsharpness
U_d^2 = detector unsharpness
U_m^2 = motion unsharpness

Noise

The radiographic *noise* or *mottle* is the random fluctuation of film density about some mean value, following uniform exposure. Noise degrades image quality and limits the ability to visualize low-contrast objects or lesions. Radiographic noise is mainly divided as follows:
○ Quantum mottle
○ Screen-film mottle.

The random variation in X-ray intensity is known as *mottle*, since it gives grainy appearance. This is due to random variations of X-ray photons that are incident on the detector, which is known as quantum mottle. This depends on the concentration of X-ray photons. Quantum mottle can be reduced by increasing the number X-ray photons reaching the detector. This will make invisible lesion into visible, but contrast is unchanged. Quantum mottle is the most important source of noise in radiography. The adjacent areas of the film receive photons that differ from the mean value, which contribute to quantum mottle. The number of X-ray photons required to produce an image is about 10^5 per mm². Whereas, in light photography, photons of 10^9 per mm² is used, hence, the noise is very low. Quantum mottle can be analyzed with **Poisson statistics**. Screen-film mottle is further divided into:

Screen-film Image Quality, Artifacts and Quality Assurance

- Screen mottle
- Film mottle
- Quantum mottle.

The screen mottle is caused by nonuniformities in screen construction (grain size), but usually negligible in modern screens. Film noise is caused by the grain structure of emulsions, which has very little concern in radiography. Quantum mottle is the major contributor in screen-film noise. It is created by the statistical fluctuations in the number of photons (quanta) per unit area, absorbed by the intensifying screen. To increase the screen-film speed, thicker screens are recommended. Such screens are called *fast screens* and absorb same number of X-rays as that of thinner screen. The image mottle of the thicker screen remains the same in such a system.

If N is the mean number of X-rays recorded by a pixel in a detector, then noise (σ) = $\sqrt{N}$, where σ is the standard deviation, which indicates photon fluctuation. Usually, Poisson statistics is used to quantify quantum noise. In this statistics, the mean (N) is equal to variance (σ^2). The relative noise, or coefficient of variation (COV) = σ/N. As the number of photons (N) increases, the relative noise decreases. As per the statistics, 68% of the regions may contain within one standard deviation (σ). Similarly, 95% and 99% of the region may lie within 2σ and 3σ, respectively.

The inverse of the relative noise is called signal-to-noise ratio (SNR), hence,

$$SNR = N/\sigma = N/\sqrt{N} = \sqrt{N}$$

To increase the SNR, the number of photons (N) reaching the detector has to be increased. As the photon number increases, the relative standard deviation decreases, and the noise is reduced. If the X-ray tube emits 100 photons, the standard deviation is 10 and the relative standard deviation is 10%. If the number of photons is increased to 1000, the standard deviation is 100 and the relative standard deviation is only 1%. This will result in reduction of noise. But it increases the patient dose, hence, optimal balance of SNR and radiation dose is a must. The detector does not detect all the incident photons. The screen-film system detects only 60% of the incident X-ray photons.

To quantify noise *Wiener spectrum* (WS) is used. It is a measure of total noise recorded by the film. Later, the film is scanned by a microdensitometer and density fluctuations is analyzed. The spectrum plots the noise of the system as a function of frequency content. Low and high frequency noise can easily be identified. The acceptable frequency range is 0.2–1 lp/mm. The Weiner spectrum can be related to MTF, photon number (N) and film gamma (G) as follows:

$$WS = \frac{G^2}{N} \times MTF^2$$

Fluoroscopy Noise

Fluoroscopy system uses image intensifier tube with TV system or flat panel systems. Only few number of X-ray photons are used to form a single frame in fluoroscopy. Radiography employs 100 times, more number of X-ray photons. Hence, quantum mottle is greater in fluoroscopy. Fluoroscopy mottle is 10 times higher compared with radiography. In the case of mammography verses fluoroscopy, the number of incident photons (air kerma) vary drastically. Hence, the noise also varies accordingly in both the systems. Fluoro image appears more noisy than mammography image.

Geometric Factors

Production of X-ray image requires proper exposure and intensity, which depends on number of geometric factors, that affects the image quality, as follows:
- Magnification
- Penumbra
- Focal spot blur.

Magnification

All radiographic images are magnified and the magnification (M) is the ratio between the image size and object size. This means that, all images are larger than their object size. Magnification is desired in some procedures, which is called magnification radiography. Generally, majority of radiographic examination needs minimum magnification. Magnification can be quantified as *magnification factor* (MF), it is the ratio of the given image size to object size. In a clinical set up, measurement of object size is difficult, hence, distance ratio is used. If SID is the source to image distance and SOD is the source to object distance, then;

$$MF = SID/SOD$$

When the object is closer to the source, the magnification is larger (Figs. 6.5A and B). When the object moves away from the source,

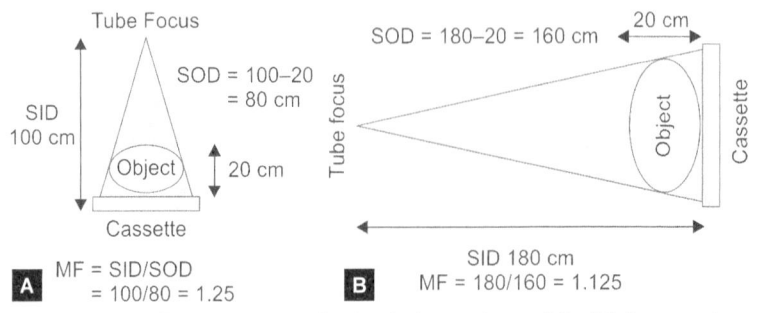

Figs. 6.5A and B: (A) The magnification higher at shorter SID; (B) Compared to higher SID.

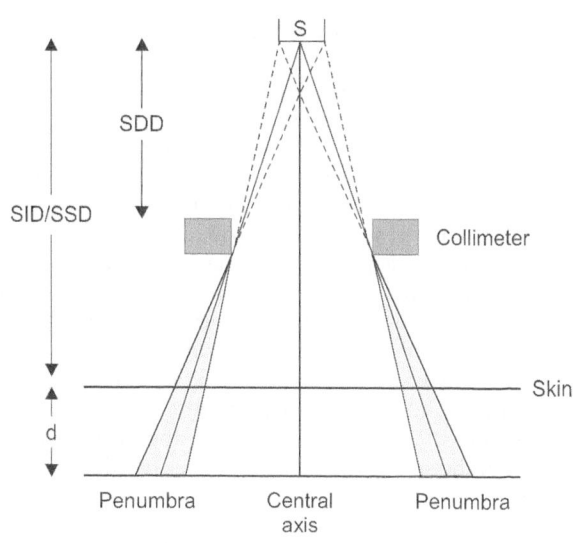

Screen-film Image Quality, Artifacts and Quality Assurance

Fig. 6.6: Geometric penumbra.

magnification decreases. This is true for the objects positioned in the central beam, as well as in lateral to central beam, for a given SID.

To minimize magnification, one can have large SID, by keeping the object very close to the receptor as much as possible. For chest radiography, the SOD is about 180 cm, and the magnification is nearly unity (about 1.05). In abdomen radiography, the SOD is 100 cm and the MF is usually, about 1.1. Lesser is the magnification means, image blur is less and higher is the resolution.

Penumbra

Penumbra is a region at the edge of a radiation beam, in which the dose rate changes as a function of distance from the beam axis (Fig. 6.6). There are three types of penumbra namely; *geometrical penumbra, transmission penumbra and physical penumbra*. The penumbra at a depth below the skin surface P_d is mainly due to geometry of the source, which is given by the relation:

$$P_d = \frac{s(SSD + d - SDD)}{SDD}$$

where, s is the source diameter, SSD or SID is the source to surface/image distance, d is the depth below the surface and SDD is the source to diaphragm distance. The penumbra increases with increase in SSD, source size and depth, but decreases with an increase in SDD. The above penumbra is a geometrical penumbra. Though the penumbra depth is increased by geometry, its width of the penumbra region depends on scattering of both collimator and patient. Transmission penumbra is caused by the beam passing through part of the collimator.

Geometrical penumbra is present both inside and outside the geometrical bounties of the beam. It is responsible for the dose fall off at the beam edges. However, reduced scatter due to transmission penumbra (collimator) also contribute to the dose fall off at the edges. In addition, scattering from patient/phantom also contribute to the dose reduction at the edges. Hence, geometric penumbra alone is not sufficient to measure beam sharpness near the edges. Therefore, the concept of **physical penumbra** is used. It accounts the overall effect of geometry, transmission penumbra, including patient/phantom scattering.

For an ideal X-ray beam, the penumbra should be at minimum and it is possible with a point source. However, in practice finite sources are used, where the focus size is large resulting in appreciable penumbra. It is also known that the size of the penumbra does not depend on the size of the radiation field.

Focal Spot Blur

The focal spot (F) of an X-ray tube is not a point and have a dimension (0.6–1.8 mm), which produce penumbra at the edges of the field. Penumbra is the region at the edges, where the radiation intensity decreases laterally, as stated above. It causes blurred region at the field edges in a radiograph, which is called focal spot blur (f):

$$f = F(M-1)$$

The focal spot blur increases with large focal spot size and higher magnification. It is small on the anode side and large on the cathode side, due to *Heel effect*. To reduce blur, smaller focal spot size and lesser magnification should be used. To have lesser magnification, the patient-film distance is reduced by keeping them close to each other.

Imaging System Performance

Overall, the diagnostic performance of the system must be good. That means the system should maximize *true positive* and *true negative* results. True positive are positive test results in patients, who have the disease. True negative are negative results in patients, who have no disease. In a similar way, *false positive* refers positive results for patients with no disease and *false negative* for negative results for patients with disease.

Imaging system should have *sensitivity* and *specificity*. The former is the ability to detect a disease, also called *true–positive fraction*. A most sensitive system will have low false negative results. Specificity is the ability of the system to identify absence of disease, also called *true-negative fraction*. This type of system should have low false-positive results. To compare the performance of an imaging system, *receiver operating*

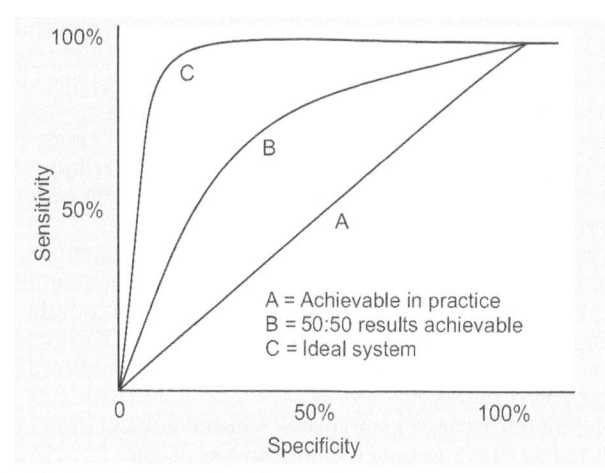

Fig. 6.7: Receiver operating characteristic curve of the imaging system.

characteristic curve (ROC) is employed. It is a curve drawn between the sensitivity in Y-axis and specificity in X-axis. The area under the curve is a measure of performance of the an imaging system (Fig. 6.7).

Optimal Quality Image

Radiographs with good quality images can be produced with proper patient preparation, selection of imaging devices and correct exposure techniques.

The patient anatomy should be placed closer to the receptor/film. The axis of the anatomy should lie parallel to the receptor plane. The central X-ray beam should pass through the center of the anatomical region. If multiple anatomies are to be imaged with equal magnification, then all the anatomical structures must be positioned at equal distance from the film. The patient must be immobilized to avoid motion blur. Motion blur can be reduced by the following:

- Short exposure time
- Providing instructions to the patient
- Keeping the source to image distance higher
- Keeping the object to image distance smaller.

Selection of exposure technique plays an important role in obtaining a good quality image. The exposure time should be always shorter, which will improve image quality. Shorter exposure time reduces motion blur. High frequency generator provides short exposure time, than single phase generators.

The kVp controls the radiographic contrast, since it influences both quantity and quality of X-rays. As the kVp increases, higher amount of

X-rays are transmitted through the patient. It reaches the film and affects the OD. Compton interaction also increases, differential absorption is reduced, resulting in reduction of subject contrast. The scatter radiation that reaches the film is higher, which increases noise in the image, resulting in loss of contrast. As the contrast is low, the latitude is larger and the margin of error is increased. Hence, high kVp reduces contrast and the only advantage is the reduction of patient dose with wide latitude of exposures.

The mA controls OD of the film, since it influences quantity of X-rays. As the mA increases, the number of X-rays reaching the film increases, resulting in higher OD. The radiographic noise is lower, but the patient dose is higher. Too low mA and high mA shift the OD away from the straight line portion of the characteristic curve. Thus, it indirectly affects the radiographic contrast.

Therefore, always use high kVp with reduced mA and short exposure time; it is the way for best quality radiographic images.

Distortion

Distortion is result of unequal magnification of different parts of an object. It may be caused by *object thickness (size), object position*, and *object shape*. Size distortion gives increased image size, compared to its original size. The SID and SOD have much role to reduce size distortion. Anatomical parts having higher object to image distance (OID) will always have higher distortion of this type. Thick objects produce unequal magnification, results in more distortion than thin objects.

Patient with irregular anatomy may contribute to distortion in a radiograph. Shape distortion may appear in two ways: *Elongation* and *foreshortening*. In elongation, the image appear longer than the true object. In foreshortening, the image appears shorter than the true. Shape distortion often occurs due to inaccurate alignment of X-ray beam center, object and detector. This type of distortion is useful for interpretation of images in few patients.

If the object plane and imaging plane are not parallel then distortion occurs, due to positioning. The distortion is minimal for object that is positioned at the center. Object that is positioned lateral to the center may have severe distortion. The objects that are lateral may have unequal magnification than that at the center. The angle of inclination of the object also influences the degree of distortion. Distorted radiographic image always have reduction in spatial resolution.

Reciprocity Failure

The reciprocity law states that, the optical density (OD) produced on a radiograph is proportional only to the total energy imported to the X-ray film and independent of the exposure time. In other words, the total exposure is not proportional to time, but proportional to the product of

Screen-film Image Quality, Artifacts and Quality Assurance

X-ray intensity (tube current in mA) and time (s), that is in mAs. That means, whether it is short or long exposure, the OD will be the same, if the given mAs is constant. This can be given as $E = It$, where E is the exposure, I is the intensity, and t is the time. This means that E is a constant, whatever the combination of I and t is. But this is true only for direct exposure of films, not true for screen-film systems.

In the case of screen-film combination, the above law fails and the total exposure is proportional to time (s). Very long or very short exposure time results in density values that are less than the expected. This means that use of very high mA and short exposure times, or very low mA and long exposure times, will not give the same density. This is known as *reciprocity failure* as stated by **Abney**. Reciprocity law failure is significant at <0.1 ms or >2 s of exposure time. The OD is lesser at such low and high exposure times. The reciprocity law is very important for special procedures, e.g. angiography (short exposure) and mammography (long exposure). Different films have different reciprocity characteristics.

ARTIFACTS

A good quality radiograph is very important for clinical diagnosis. Whenever the quality of radiograph is not satisfactory, it is important to discover the cause, for preventing this mistake in future. The cause need not be from the darkroom, it can be from elsewhere also. The following summary gives the defects and the possible causes (Tables 6.1 and 6.2) (Figs. 6.8A to D).

QUALITY ASSURANCE

Sensitometry

Sensitometry is a photographic science, introduced by **Hurter and Driffield**. It tells about the evaluation of the performance of photographic material, e.g. X-ray film. In this, the X-ray film is exposed to a specified light source or X-ray source for fixed times and then the emulsion is processed under standard conditions. The resultant densities produced on the film are then measured and graphed versus a logarithmic scale of radiation exposure. Hence, sensitometry is basically the study of relationship between the radiation exposure and film density. It is very much useful to study the characteristics of the film and screen-film combinations in medicine. It can also be used to evaluate the automatic film processor. The various equipment used for the above purpose are:
- Penetrometer
- Sensitometer.

Characteristic curve is drawn by having density on the vertical axis (Y) and log of exposure in the horizontal axis (X). It can be produced by the following methods:

Medical X-ray Film Processing

Table 6.1: General defects and causes in manual film processing.

Type of artifact	Causes
1. Inadequate general blackening	Under exposure/Developing time too short/Insufficiently replenished developer/Developing time not adjusted to the temperature of the path/Bad composition of the developer.
2. Excessive general blackening	Overexposure/Overlong developing time/Developing time not adjusted to the temperature of the path/Bad composition of the developer.
3. Excessive contrast	Oversoft rays (too low kV) when taking radiograph/Developing time too long/Bad composition of the developer bath.
4. Inadequate contrast	Overharsh rays (too high kV) when taking radiograph/Overexposure compensated for by shorter developing time/Too short developing time for the temperature of the bath/Exhausted developer bath/Unsuitable or wrongly prepared developer.
5. Insufficient sharpness	Too short focus-film distance/Vibration of the X-ray tube or movement by patient during the radiograph/Overlarge or damaged focus/Patient not sufficiently pressed against cassette or film/Bad contact between film and screen/Insufficient sharpness (owing to over coarse grain) of the intensifying screens/Influence of secondary rays.
6. Gray fog	Darkroom lighting not in order/Film exposed to darkroom light for too long or held too close to the lamp/Influence of undesirable X-rays or white light/Film too old or stored in bad conditions/Salts in the developer. The loaded cassette exposed too long to excessive heat/Film examined too quickly in white light during the fixing/Inadequate closing of the cassette/Bad composition of the developer.
7. Yellow fog	Prolonged developing time in oxidized developer (solution turned very brown)/Exhausted bath/Inadequate fixing.
8. Chemical or dichroic fog (yellowish-green by reflected light and pink by transmitted light)	Developer contaminated by fixing bath/Inadequate rinsing after development and exhausted fixing bath/Prolonged developing time in exhausted bath/Film exposed to white light during the fixing, while exhausted fixing bath is used.
9. Streaky gray fog	Film too old or incorrectly stored.
10. White precipitation	Inadequate intermediate rinsing when using the hardening fixing bath.

Contd...

Contd...

Type of artifact	Causes
11. Light spots	Air bubbles (very small, sharply-delineated spots): Film insufficiently agitated during the first 30 seconds in the developer/Drops of fixing or stop-bath fell on the film before it was placed in the developer/Impression of sharp objects on the film, the packing or the container. If this happens before the exposure, then the spots are brighter than their surroundings/Dry spots over rapid or irregular drying, causing drops by collection of water. The films stuck together or to the wall of the tank during development. Greasy spots on the film prevent the developer from penetrating the emulsion/defective intensifying screens/Impurities between intensifying screen and film. Small pitted spots, in most cases with dark edges: Influence of bacteria. Too slow drying in a hot damp climate, especially if the washing water is not very pure.
12. Light lines or streaks	Writing on the envelope before exposure/Insufficient agitation during the development process/Irregular drying/Drops of fixing or spot-bath run over the emulsion before the development process.
13. Light marks	Moon-shaped: Cracking of film caused by taking hold of it with more than two fingers prior to exposure/Fingerprints: Film touched before development by fingers which are too greasy or soiled with fixing bath or stop-bath, some other acid.
14. Dark spots	Drops of developer bath on the film prior to developing/Drops of water on the film before development/Static charge as a result of friction in fairly dry air/Impression of sharp objects on the film after exposure/Irregular drying. Damp patches remaining on the film when it is removed from the drying cabinet/Small pieces of metal stuck to the film during the development process.
15. Dark lines or streaks	Scratches on the emulsion after exposure/Impression of sharp objects after exposure of film/Insufficient agitation during development/Irregular drying/Drops of developer or water ran down the film prior to the developing process.
16. Dark marks	Moon-shaped. Bending the film as result of taking of it with more than two fingers after exposure/Fingerprints: Film taken hold of prior to development with fingers soiled with developer/Small bush-shaped marks as a result of electrostatic charge.
17. Yellow stain	Prolonged development in old, oxidized developer/Inadequate intermediate rinsing/Exhausted fixing bath.
18. Brown patches	Improper fixing/Diluted fixer/Exhausted fixer/Lack of agitation in fixer.
19. Blue-green stains	Exhausted fixer/High temperature of fixer.

Contd...

Contd...

Type of artifact	Causes
20. Metallic appearance	Deposition of oxidation produced on the film.
21. Mottle and streaks	Lack of agitation in developer/fixer retained in hangers.
22. Reticulation	Extreme temperature variation in successive processing tank.
23. Crescent-shaped black mark (kink mark)	Local sharp bend handling.
24. Water marks	Film left to dry in hangers.
25. Black circular spots	Film left to dry before development.
26. White circular spots	Splash of fixer before development.
27. Branching, radiating or tree-like marks	Charging friction or pressure between film and interleaf or intensifying screen.
28. Clustered white spots	Dust or foreign substances on intensifying screen.

Defects—During development

Type of artifact	Causes
29. Lighter or darker streaks	Insufficient agitation during the development process. This defect occurs especially in sectors which contrast sharply with the upper zones. It is caused by the fact that bromide increases locally the specific weight of the solution and runs down the emulsion.
30. Fog	Effect of undesirable lighter in the darkroom/Overlong or overclose exposure to darkroom light/Copper, tin, etc., salts in the developer. In this case, the fog thickens if the film is often removed from the bath and if the air is warm.
31. Yellowish or dichroic fog	Bath in use too long/Overlong developing time/Excessive temperature of the bath/Contamination of the developer bath by the fixing bath.

Defects—During fixing

Type of artifact	Causes
32. Gray-brown spots or streaks	Inadequate fixing. This failure is mostly due to the action of light on unresolved silver halides.
33. Blurred image	This happens only infrequently in the case of negatives.
34. Yellow fog	Exhausted alkaline or silvery fixing bath.
35. White spots	Inadequate agitation (these spots can be removed by means of aqueous solution of sodium carbonate (10%).

Defects due to insufficient rinsing

Type of artifact	Causes
36. Films insufficiently rinsed	Too much developer passes into the fixing bath, which means that: ➢ The fixing bath becomes alkaline too quickly (increase in the pH value). ➢ White spots can occur if a developer with strong alkaline is used and subsequently a hardening fixing bath with aluminum salt.

Screen-film Image Quality, Artifacts and Quality Assurance

Table 6.2: Faults in automatic film processing.

(i) Processing faults:

1. Longitudinal scratches	This is connected with guide plates in the racks. Remove the processor lid and override the cut-out switch.
2. Pipe lines	This is caused by chemicals partially drying out on rollers. This will be repeated intervals equal to the diameter of the roller.
3. White or black spots	This is caused by breakdown on the surface of a hard roller. Sometimes this will resemble calculi or phleboliths, leads to wrong diagnosis. Each roller has to be checked.
4. Drying marks	This can be seen only in reflected light, appear as dull longitudinal lines. These are caused by dirt or dust blocking part of the air knife.
5. Nondrying marks	It is due to the fault in the fixer. Measure pH and silver levels in the fixer and check replenisher pumps.

(ii) General faults:

6. High density marks	Black splashes: They appear as splash on the film. The reason is that the film has been splashed with developer/water before development, splash area develops faster than surrounding area, causing high density. Black marks: These are in various shapes namely crescent shaped and black fingerprints. The former is caused by bad film handling techniques. Technician gripping the film tightly between thumb and forefinger. The latter is caused by technician who has developer/water on his hands. *Static marks*: This marks looks exactly like the branches of a tree. The causes are (i) formica type bench and vinyl floor— cover the bench with oil based linoleum. ➢ Dry atmosphere in the darkroom. ➢ Technician wearing nylon fabric. ➢ Loading and unloading of film into the cassette— screen needs to be cleaned regularly.
7. Surface marks	These are single-sided and appear in the surface of the film. Algae in the wash tank, bits of emulsion in developer, fixer and wash tank. Check the tank and clean it.
8. Pressure marks	Can be white or black, appear randomly over the film. Incorrect film storage or poor film handling. Check handling and storage.
9. Radiation or light fogging	Randomly appear and cover larger areas. If the film is fogged through a material, then faint image of the material will be seen. This is due to fogging by radiation. The black marks around the edge of the film are due to light leakage in the cassette or the film box is opened in daylight.

Contd...

Medical X-ray Film Processing

Contd...

10. Overall high density	This is caused by lead based paint, varnishes, formaldehyde, carbon monoxide, mercury (not to use Hg thermometer), developer (films and chemicals not to be stored in the same room), heat (maintain 20°C), time of storage (check shelf life), incorrect safe light (check bulb wattage, filter and for cracks in the filter) and background radiation.
11. Low density marks	This is due to (i) fixer splashed on to the film before development, the splash area is cleared before development and appears as white, (ii) grease or oil on the surface of the film through technician's hand.
12. White marks	This will be in the form of (i) crescent shaped due to bad handling before exposure, (ii) white fingerprints caused by fixer or oil in technician's hand, and (iii) pressure marks.
13. Sharply defined marks	This is due to artifacts inside the cassette. Artifact in the screen reduces light output to the film and hence, white marks appear. Developer, fixer, and water can damage intensifying screens. Physical damage to screen (scratches) also can create white marks.

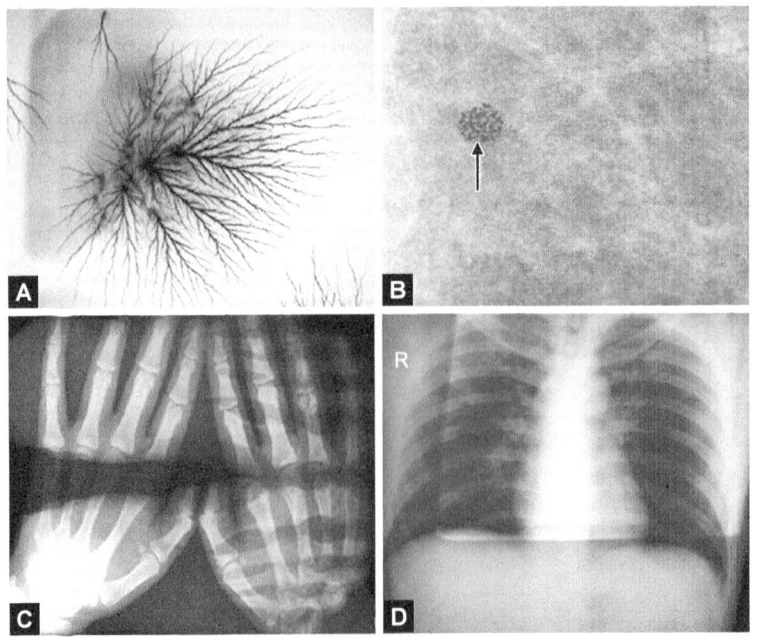

Figs. 6.8A to D: Radiography artifacts: Manual film processing (A) static artifact and (B) water stain artifact. Automatic film processing: (C) double exposure artifact and (D) scattering fog artifact.

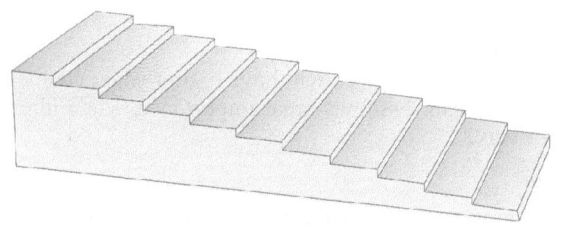

Screen-film Image Quality, Artifacts and Quality Assurance

Fig. 6.9A: Penetrometer.

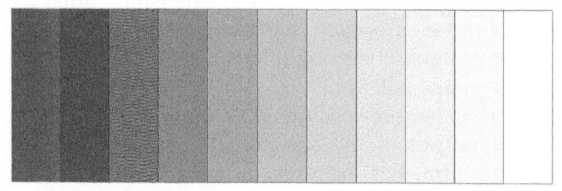

Fig. 6.9B: Image of a step wedge exposed to X-rays on a film, revealing full range of densities from black to light gray or white.

- Time scale sensitometry
- Intensity scale of sensitometry
- Penetrometer.

In time scale sensitometry, kV, mA and distance are kept constant and the time of exposure is varied, by a factor of 2. The first part exposed will receive the highest exposure and the last part will have the least. Eleven exposures (21 is ideal) are sufficient to plot the characteristic curve. In intensity scale sensitometry, kV distance and time are kept constant and mA is varied. Other procedure is similar to the first method.

A penetrometer or step wedge is a device of uniform absorbers of increasing thickness, made up of aluminum or tissue equivalent plastic (Fig. 6.9A). The step wedge is kept on a film and exposed to X-rays. It will produce uniform densities that resemble a step wedge (Fig. 6.9B). This wedge should have a copper layer on the base to create homogeneous beam. The wedge has to be calibrated precisely, so that each step on the wedge produces an exact and regular increase or decrease in exposure.

Opacity and Density

When standard light is passed through the X-ray film, the ratio of the incident and transmitted light is termed as opacity, i.e.

$$\text{Opacity} = \frac{\text{Incident light}}{\text{Transmitted light}}$$

The log of the opacity is called density. It defines the amount of blackening on the film. For example, if 10 light photons are transmitted out of 100 incident photons then,

Opacity = 100/10 = 10
Density = log 10 = 1

Films with higher densities will have higher silver content per unit area. Hence, this factor assumes great importance, when films are sold for silver recovery.

Sensitometer

A sensitometer is a device that exposes a film to a range of known, constant light intensities having proper light wavelength sensitivity. It is capable of producing consistent step wedge densities. It has a controlled light source to expose an optical step wedge template. The step wedge template transmits light of varying intensities on the film. Once the film is processed, the image will appear as density step wedge.

It merely simulates, the spectral emission of the intensifying screens used. The light output of the sensitometer must match the spectral sensitivity of the film. For example, a green light sensitometer is to be used with a green sensitive film. It is wrong to use a blue emitting sensitometer with an orthochromatic film (green). Sensitometers exist in many forms, from simple three-patch sensitometers to large 21-step negative for printing.

A typical sensitometer is shown in Figure 6.10. It has a calibrated light filter which provides about 20 different light intensities to expose the film. The given film is loaded in the sensitometer in the darkroom. Now, the film is exposed to range of light intensities that are matched to

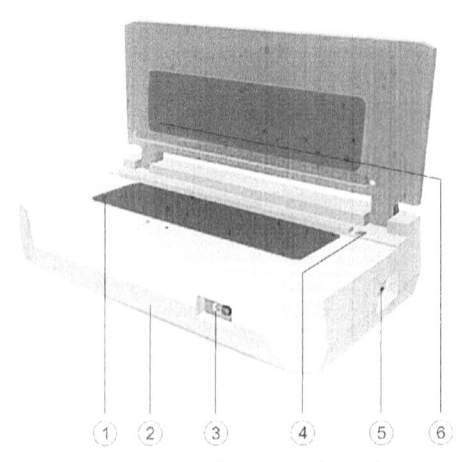

Fig. 6.10: Sensitometer. (1) Window with step wedge, (2) Sticker with type and serial number (at the bottom), (3) Switch for sensitivity (blue or green sensitive films), (4) Button for exposure (will be activated by pressing down the cover), (5) Input for external power supply, and (6) Cover.
(*Courtesy:* PTW Dosimetry India Pvt. Ltd.)

Screen-film Image Quality, Artifacts and Quality Assurance

the wavelength sensitivity of the film. Then the film is developed in the processor which is to be tested. The final film will have differing density, known as *sensitometry strip*. This strip is introduced in the densitometer and the corresponding density values are measured.

Densitometer

A densitometer is a device that measures the amount of incident light transmitted through the developed film. If I_0 is the incident light, It is the transmitted light then OD = $\log_{10}(I_0/I_t)$. As the transmitted light decreases in dark areas of the film, the OD gets increased. It is mainly used to read the relative density of the various steps on the sensitometry strip (film). If the OD of the sensitometric strip is plotted on semilogarithmic paper, the characteristic curve will appear. The curve demonstrates the relationship between radiation exposure (X-axis) and density (Y-axis). The position of the curve on the X-axis and its shape depend on the given radiographic film.

It measures the quantity of light, passing through the step wedge area. The density can either be read directly, or seen as light-emitting diode (LED) display for each step. With the OD and log of exposure values, the characteristic curve can be plotted by hand. Modern densitometers are linked with computer, which can automatically read density and print the characteristic curve for the film. The above information can be stored and weekly printouts are obtained. With densitometer, one can assess the processor activities and also compare different processors.

A typical densitometer is shown in Figure 6.11. From the densitometer measurements, one can obtain base + fog density, mid-density level

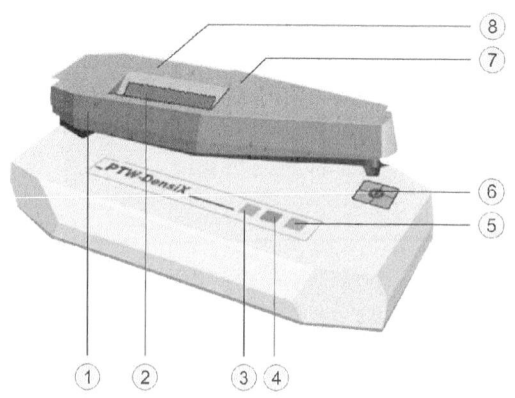

Fig. 6.11: Densitometer. (1) Measuring arm, (2) LC display, (3) Button on/Next for switching on and toggling (next measurement, varies values and functions), (4) Button Zero for zero-processing, (5) Button off to switch off DensiX LE, (6) Measuring area, (7) Sticker with type and serial number (at the bottom), and (8) Socket for external power supply (rear).
(*Courtesy*: PTW Dosimetry India Pvt. Ltd.)

(OD close to 1.0 above base + fog level), density difference between 0.25 and 2.0 above base + fog level, respectively. Once a particular step is identified, they can be used in next day measurements. The base + fog reading helps us to conclude whether the film is unduly exposed to background radiation, harsh conditions or improper processing. Higher value of base + fog will offset the film contrast and image quality. The mid-density level determines the speed of the film and variations caused by processing conditions. The density difference determines the consistency of the film response and processing. Thus, densitometer measurements trace the trends and establish control limits of processor performance.

7

Digital Radiography

DIGITAL SYSTEMS

Digital Basics

Digital radiography is a field in which digital detectors are used, instead of X-ray film. It produces digital images, instead of an analog image. Hence, screen-film systems are replaced by digital radiography systems. Digital images have the following advantages:
O Data can be stored and transferred
O It allows image post processing
O Display of images in computer monitor
O Use of picture archiving and communication systems (PACS) for Tele-radiology.

Computers use binary system for which the base is 2. The value of a digit in a position is 2 times, than its in right and no decimal is allowed. We have been using decimal system in which the left digit is 10 times higher than its right. The term *binary digit (bit)* is the basic element used in digital system. One bit can be assigned either one of the discrete values; 0 or 1. Similarly, bit can be assigned gray shades either white or block.

In general, computer memory and storage use many bits and each bit has two states, namely 0 or 1. Similarly, 2 bit may have 4 possible state, 3 bits have 8 states and so on. In general, if there are N bits than the possible states are 2^N, e.g. 8 bit may have 2^8 states, which is equal to 258 gray shades. However, radiography involves large field size and a resolution of about 10 lp/mm, to provide optimal contrast. Therefore, it requires higher bit depth of 8, 12 and 16, respectively. For example, 16 bit depth can provide 65, 536 numbers of gray shades. That is why digital radiography needs large storage space in the range of 4-32 MB, which is very much higher, compared to a computed tomography scanner.

Additional terms like *byte* and *word* are used in digital systems. One byte = 8 bits and one word = 2 bytes or 16 bits. Additionally, kilobyte (kB), megabyte (MB), gigabyte (GB) and terabyte (TB) are also used:
O 2^{10} = 1024 byte = 1 kB
O 20^{20} = 1048 kB = 1 MB
O 20^{30} = 1073 MB = 1 GB
O 20^{40} = 1024 GB = 1 TB.

Computer Basics

A typical computer has the following components:
O Central Processing Unit (CPU)
O Memory

- Data entry
- Export device.

Computer memory stores various bit values, either in random access memory (RAM) or read only memory (ROM). A *RAM* is a temporary memory, whereas ROM is a permanent memory. CPU instructions are stored in the *ROM*. In addition, there are buffer and cache memories. The former is used in video display, and the later performs as a buffer in between RAM and memory disk. Basically, computers are operated with software systems, which can store files. An operating system is a software, which acts as an interface between the user and computer hardware. Such operating systems are as follows:

- Windows (Microsoft)
- Mac OS, iOS (Apple)
- UNIX
- Android OS (Goggle)
- VMS (Main frame computer).

Computer programs are written using the following languages:

- C, C++
- COBOL
- FORTRON
- Java, Java script
- Pythan
- Pascal.

Computer employs lot of peripheral devices in the form of input and output devices as given below:

Input devices
- Mouse
- Key board
- Joy stick
- Light pen
- Track ball
- Touch screen
- Scanner
- Digitizer
- Microphone.

Output devices
- Monitor (LED,LCD,CRT)
- Printer
- Projector
- Plotter
- Audio speaker
- Head phones.

Data storage devices
- Hand drive
- CD-ROM
- DVD-ROM
- Flash media
- Thumb drive
- Memory stick
- iPOD
- Digital camera.

Computer is connected via co-axial cable, telephone lines, magnetic tape transfer, microwave and fiber-optics. A *modem* is used to transfer data through telephone lines. Cable modem is used to transfer data in cable television lines. The data transfer rate (per second) is called *Baud rate*. To connect modem computers network is used, e.g. *Ethernet*.

Digital Image Format

A digital image is divided into number of rows and columns, called *matrix*. The matrix sizes are 128 × 128 (Gamma camera), 256 × 256 (MRI), 512 × 512 (CT, US), 1024 × 1024 (DSA), 2560 × 2048 (CR, DR) and 4096 × 6144 (Mammography). The smallest element in the matrix is called *pixel*. It stands for picture element in 2D image. This is seen in TV monitor or in hard copy print out. But, patient anatomy is in 3D and a discrete value called *voxel* is used. It stands for volume element in a patient. Hence, a pixel (2D) in the monitor represents an voxel (3D) in the patient. A pixel size is the ratio of *field of view* (FOV) and the matrix size. Typical pixel sizes used in radiology ranges from 0.5–1 mm.

While viewing a digital image, each pixel is assigned a value, related to signal intensity. The value stored in the pixel is in binary format and the maximum value that is stored is called *bit depth*. A pixel having a high value represents dark gray shade, whereas pixel of low value represents white gray shade. This is analogy with film, where high dose gives dark shade and low dose gives white shade. A single bit can store either, black or white, similar to an electrical switch, which can be switched ON or OFF.

Digital Detector Systems

Digital systems use the following detectors, to produce radiological image:
- Gas detector
- Solid state detector.

Gas detectors are basically ionization chamber and contain air or special gases. When exposed to X-rays, ion pairs are produced in the gas. These ion pairs are collected by applying an electric field between the electrodes. Thus, measurement of ionization current creates an electrical signal. The total charge collected is proportional to the radiation intensity. Detectors in imaging uses gases of high Z at high pressure, e.g. Xenon (Z = 54).

Solid state detector consists of inner and outer energy bands such as valance and conduction bands. When the detector is exposed to X-rays, valance band electrons absorb energy by Compton and photoelectric process. These electrons move to the conduction band and form electron traps, just below the conduction band. In some phosphor, the electrons return to the ground state instantaneously, with emission of light. Some phosphors require light/heat stimulation to return the electrons to the ground state with emission of light. Such a emission of light is called *luminescence*. Solid state detectors come in the following category:
- Scintillator detector
- Photoconductor detector
- Photostimulable phosphor detector.

Scintillator

In the case of scintillator, the radiation excites atoms of the phosphor and emits light flashes instantly, e.g. NaI. It can be detected by a photomultiplier tube (PMT) or photodiode, which gives an electrical signal. The detected electrical signal is proportional to the incident radiation intensity. *Gadolinium oxysulfide* (GOS) and *cesium iodide* (CsI) are used as scintillators.

Photoconductor

Photoconductor is a solid state device, e.g. *selenium* (Z = 34). When the detector is exposed to X-rays, energy is deposited and the detector emits electrons directly. The produced electron charge may be collected, by applying voltage across the photoconductor as signal. The electric charge signal is proportional to incident X-ray intensity. Since, selenium absorption is very poor, hence, *lead iodide* and *mercury iodide* are used.

Photostimulable Phosphor

Photostimulable phosphor (PSP) requires red laser light as stimulant to return the trapped electrons to the valence state, e.g. Barium fluorobromide (BaFbr). As a result, blue light is emitted, which can be measured by a PMT. The detected light intensity is proportional to the incident radiation intensity. This principle is used in imaging plates. These plates are exposed to intense white light to erase remaining electrons, so that it can be reused again. An ideal digital radiography system should have the following:
- The physical design should have compatible size with screen-film cassettes
- Immediate readout facility
- Robust and less costly
- High quantum efficiency with low radiation dose for image capture

Digital Radiography

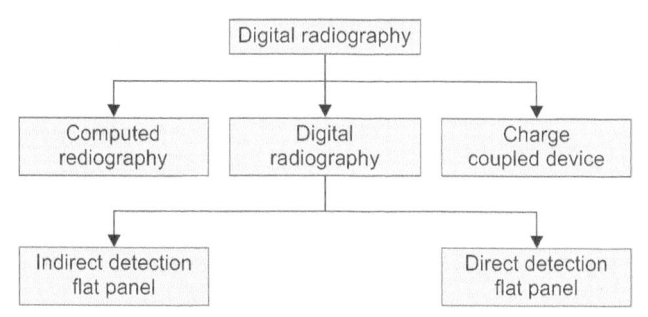

Fig. 7.1: Different path of getting digital radiography images.

- Spatial and contrast resolution similar to film
- Wide dynamic range
- Digital imaging and communications in medicine (DICOM) compatible.

Presently, these systems are employed in the following forms:
- Computed radiography (CR)
- Charge-coupled device (CCD)
- Digital radiography (DR).

The DR is further classified into indirect digital radiography and direct digital radiography (Fig. 7.1).

COMPUTED RADIOGRAPHY

Computed radiography employs a phosphor, which works on *photostimulable luminescence* (PSL) principle. When the phosphor is exposed to radiation, it absorbs and stores the radiation energy. Later, if it is stimulated by a different light source, and it gives luminescence. The amount of luminescence is proportional to incident radiation exposure.

Photostimulable Phosphor

The commonly used phosphor is *barium fluorohalides; BaFBr (85%) and BaFl (15%): Eu (europium)*. The europium is called activator and it is present in small quantity, which is responsible for the PSL property. The atomic numbers of BaFBr are 56, 9 and 35 with K-shell binding energy of 37, 5, and 12 keV, respectively. The radiation interactions are mostly by Compton and photoelectric process.

The activator creates defects in the crystals (F-center), which can trap electrons. When the phosphor is exposed to radiation, the divalent europium atoms (Eu^{+2}) get oxidized into trivalent Eu^{+3} with release of electrons in the valence band (Fig. 7.2). These electrons move from the valence band to conduction band; later they are trapped at the *F-centers* in the forbidden zone. The electrons can stay in these centers for longer

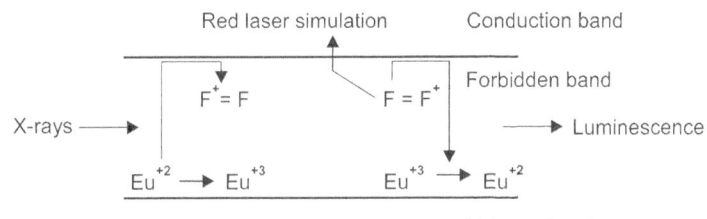

128 Medical X-ray Film Processing

Fig. 7.2: Principle of photostimulable phosphor. (Eu: europium)

period of time. Thus, billions of electrons are trapped in the F-centers. The number of electrons per unit area is proportional to the absorbed radiation energy.

$$\text{X-ray} + Eu^{+2} = Eu^{+3} + e^-$$

Over the time, these electrons may return to the ground state on their own. However, exposing the phosphor to a red light source may accelerate the electron return process. That is why, it is called photostimulable phosphor (PSP), which is used in *imaging plate* technology. When the imaging plate is scanned by *red laser light*, the F-center absorbs energy and transfers the same to the electrons. The electrons reach the conduction band, where they become mobile again. They move to the valence band, with emission of blue-green light. The electron joins with Eu^{+3} and is converted into Eu^{+2}. The *blue-green light* energy is greater than that of laser light energy.

The phosphor will not give up all its trapped electrons in the first stage of laser light. It will retain some amount of trapped electrons. Hence, it is to be exposed to very bright light source (white light), which moves all the trapped electrons to the valence band, thus emptying the F-centers is achieved. Now, the imaging plate can be used for another radiation exposure.

Imaging Plate

The phosphor can be made as flexible screen, which is enclosed in a rugged cassette and is called imaging plate (0.5 mm). Imaging plate was first introduced by **Fuji**, Japan, in 1983 and is similar to that of a screen-film cassette. The cross-section of an imaging plate is shown in Figure 7.3A. A commercial CR cassette is shown in Figure 7.3B. In the imaging plate, the PSP particles are randomly present throughout the binder and it can be handled similar to that of screen-film cassette.

The cassettes are available in various sizes, namely; 14″ × 17″, 14″ × 14″, 10″ × 12″, and 8″ × 10″ (all are in inches) with a pixel range of 200 × 200 to 100 × 100 μm. It is available in variety; for general radiography, mammography, dental, etc. The matrix sizes available are 1,760 × 2,140 for normal resolution and 2,000 × 2,510 for high resolution. The spatial

Digital Radiography   **129**

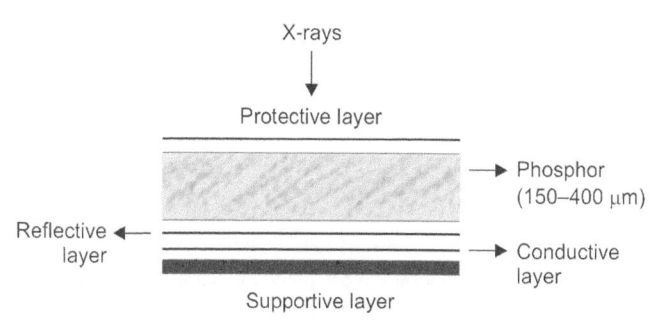

Fig. 7.3A: Cross-section of an imaging plate.

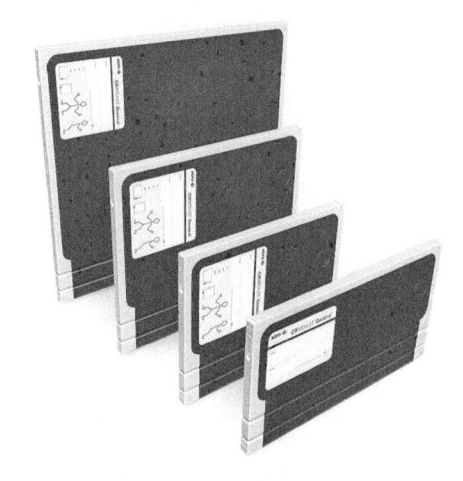

Fig. 7.3B: Commercial CR cassette of different sizes.
(*Courtesy*: M/s.Agfa Healthcare India Pvt. Ltd.)

frequency is 2–3 lp/mm for standard radiographic work, and 10 lp/mm for mammography work.

Phosphor Reader

The CR system consists of imaging plates of various sizes, a reader, computer and a printer, in addition to X-ray unit (Fig. 7.4). The computer offers image processing, storage, and image display facility. The imaging plate is used instead of screen-film cassette. It can be reused again and again by erasing old image data. The following is the procedure involved in CR:

○ Computed radiography cassette is exposed to X-ray beam
○ Cassette is inserted into the reader

130 Medical X-ray Film Processing

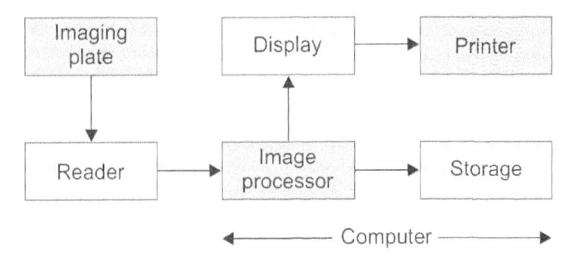

Fig. 7.4: Block diagram of computed radiography system.

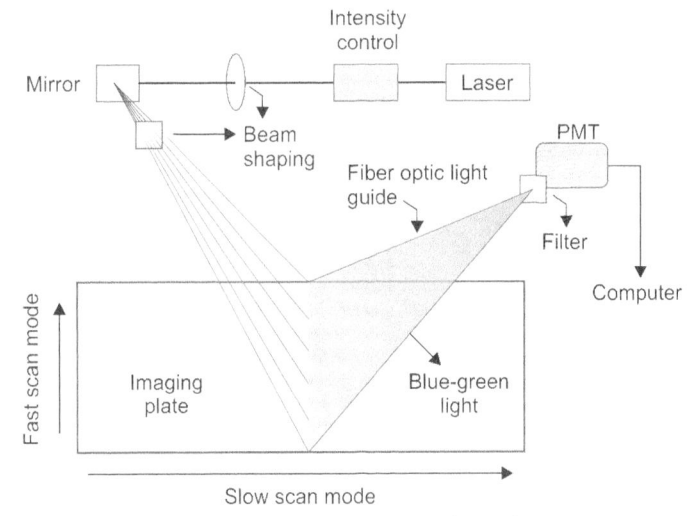

Fig. 7.5A: Computed radiography reader.
(PMT: Photomultiplier tube)

- Imaging plate is removed from the cassette
- Scanned by the He-Ne laser beam (633 nm), blue-green or UV light (390 nm) is released from that location (X, Y)
- Photomultiplier tube (PMT) is used to collect this light and gives an electronic signal
- Electronic signal is digitized and stored in memory
- The plate is exposed to bright white light, to erase the residual energy, for another use.

The reader is the most critical part of CR imaging system. The CR reader consists of an entry system for imaging plate, laser light source and a PMT (Fig. 7.5A). A typical commercial CR reader is shown in Figure 7.5B. After the radiation exposure the CR cassette is inserted into the reader, where the imaging plate is removed from the cassette and

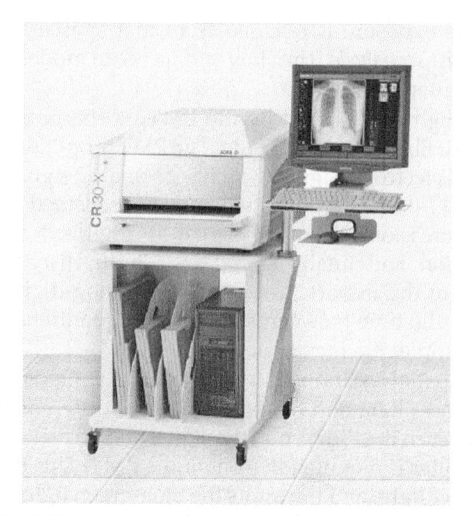

Fig. 7.5B: Commercial computed radiography system. (*Courtesy*: M/s. Agfa healthcare India Pvt. Ltd.)

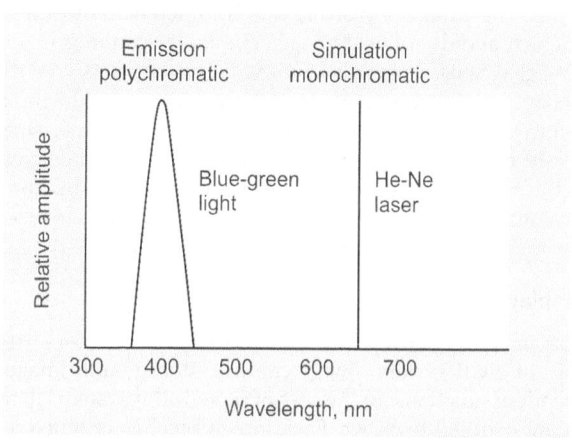

Fig. 7.6: Computed radiography spectrum: Simulation and emission of light.

fitted to a drive mechanism. The drive mechanism moves the plate with constant velocity along the Y-axis. This is usually done with slow motion and is called *slow scan mode*.

A rotating and multifaceted mirror reflects the red light from a laser source (He-Ne laser, 633 nm). This light is deflected back and forth across the phosphor plate in the horizontal, X-direction, which releases visible, blue-green light of 390 nm (Fig. 7.6). This means that the trapped energy due to radiation exposure is released from that spatial location (X, Y). This is done in *fast scan mode*. The slow and fast scan modes are controlled by the CR computer.

The above light is collected by the PMT or charge-coupled device (CCD), through a fiberoptic light guide. The PMT amplifies the signal and gives the output electronic signal, which is an analog signal varying with time. This is fed into a computer, where it is processed for amplitude, scale and compression. Then the signal is digitized with sampling and quantification and finally stored in a hard disc. Sampling and quantification are the import process in the analog-digital conversion. Sampling refers the time between samples and quantification refers the value of each sample.

For every spatial location X, Y, a grayscale value is obtained. The wavelength of laser light and blue-green light is different. The scattered laser light may reach the PMT, spoil the signal and creates noise. To avoid this, an optical filter is mounted in front of the PMT. This filter attenuates the scattered laser light, and transmits the blue-green light emitted by the phosphor, thereby increasing the signal-noise ratio.

In some other systems, the cassette is inserted vertically and imaging plate is withdrawn downward, during which it is scanned by a horizontal laser. In this, the imaging plate is not completely removed from the cassette, which avoids roller damage. The laser scanning is done right angle to the grid lines, which also avoids *aliasing artifacts*.

The laser beam size is very important and it should be kept less than 100 μm at the mirror level. The laser beam shape, size, speed, and intensity must be kept constant at the imaging plate level. This is achieved by means of a beam shaping devices. A reader can process about 70 cassettes in 1 hour and it takes about 110 seconds to process each cassette.

Image Display

The digital image is shown in the computer monitor for further post processing. In a CR system, image capture, storage and image display are independent functions. In the case of screen-film system, all the above functions are coupled together. Each image pixel is assigned a location and gray scale value. The image can be brought to the required brightness level. To do this, window level and window width can be adjusted by the user. The window level refers the center value of the window width, which control image brightness. Window width refers the range of gray scale value, which controls image contrast. Proper window width and window level achieves good brightness and image contrast. Lesser is the window width, higher the image contrast.

In the postprocessing, one can manipulate digital image data. To achieve this, tools such as *histogram equalization, low–pass spatial filter, unsharp masking, background and energy subtractions* are employed. The former eliminates the black and white pixels, since their contribution is little. This will facilitate to expand the display range. To reduce noise in the image, low-pass filter is used. In this, portion of the averaged value of the surrounding pixels is added to each pixel. Unsharp masking tool is used to subtract the smoothened version from the original. It can be added later, to resemble the original. To reduce scattered radiation, background subtraction is used, which improves image contrast.

Energy subtraction is used, where low and high kV images are obtained for a given anatomy. For example, in chest radiography bone can be subtracted, to view clearly lung and soft tissues. Alternatively, soft tissue can be filtered, to look bones clearly. This will differentiate calcified and noncalcified lung nodules. Nowadays, computer aid detection (CAD) along with artificial intelligence are used to make the diagnosis.

After postprocessing, the image is fed into a laser printer for making a hard copy. The principle and function of the printer is explained in the next chapter.

Image Characteristics

The main advantage of imaging plate is its wide dynamic range and it has wide latitude towards radiation exposure (Fig. 7.7). It can accept

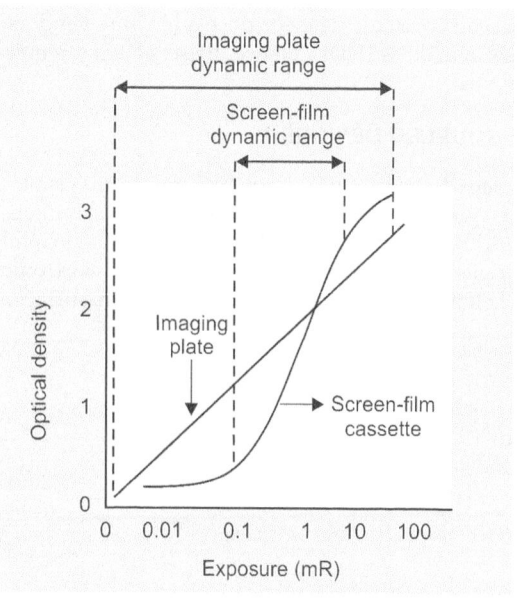

Fig. 7.7: Comparison of dynamic range of imaging plate and screen-film systems.

100 times either low or higher radiation intensities, compared to screen-film system. Usually, screen-film system requires a radiation intensity of 5 µGy for optimal image. The technologist has freedom to select his own exposure techniques (kV, mAs) in computed radiography. But technologist cannot understand his error, since it is adjusted in the image postprocessing, by window width and window level. However, the retake rate is lesser in computed radiography, compared to screen-film radiography.

The images produced with low radiation exposure, involve higher quantum noise, whereas images produced with high radiation exposure involves low noise, but involves high patient dose. The main source of noise is the scatter radiation. The drive mechanism, laser, and computer devices also contribute to noise in the image.

The CR systems are faster, compared to 400 speed screen-film system. Hence, images can be produced with lower patient dose. In screen-film radiography, kVp controls contrast and mA controls optical density, is a concept which is no more valid in CR, because CR image contrast is constant, irrespective of exposure techniques. Therefore, high kVp and lower mAs can be used to produce CR images, which reduce patient dose further.

The spatial resolution is less (3.5–5.5 lp/mm), compared to screen-film systems (8–12 lp/mm) and it is preferred in portable radiography. It is very difficult to access detector dose and some vendors came with detector dose indicators (DDI). Hence, these systems require elaborate quality assurance.

CHARGED-COUPLED DEVICES

Charge-coupled devices (CCD) form images from visible light. It is usually used with intensifying screens and image intensifier tubes (Figs. 7.8A and B). Basically, CCD chip is an integrated circuit, made up of *amorphous silicon*. Its surface is edged with pixel electronics, e.g. a 2.5 × 2.5 cm CCD may contain 1,024 × 1,024 pixels in its surface. The silicon

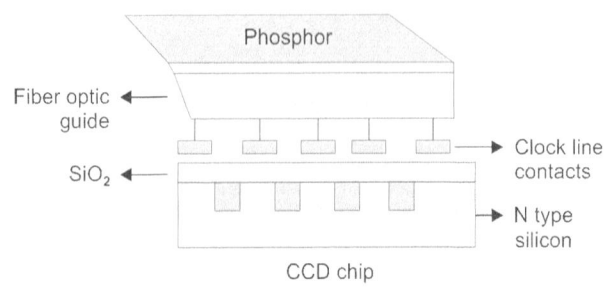

Fig. 7.8A: Design of charge-coupled device (CCD).

Digital Radiography 135

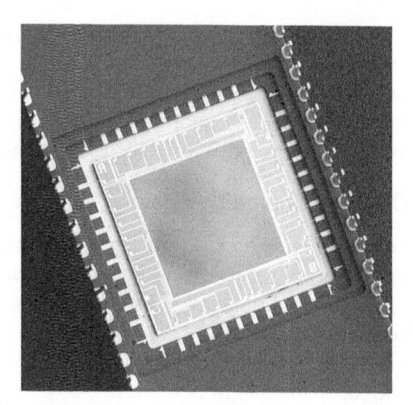

Fig. 7.8B: Typical CCD commercially available.

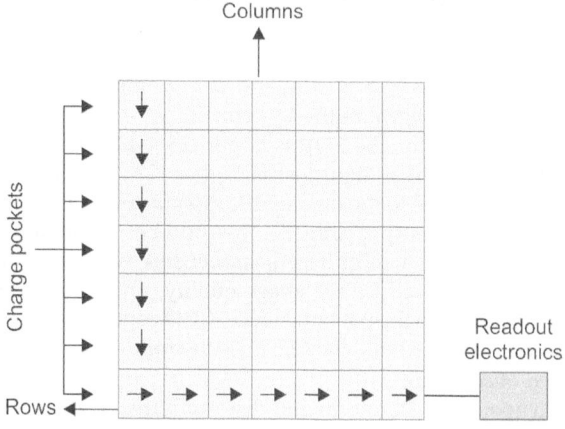

Fig. 7.9: Movement of charge pockets column-by-column through bottom row.

surface is photoconductive; if it is exposed to visible light, electrons are liberated and built up in the pixel. Higher is the light intensity, larger the electrons, that are liberated. The electrons are kept in the pixel by electronic barriers on each side of the pixel. Thus, each pixel act as capacitor and collect above charge, proportional to light.

Electronic charge in each pixel is readout along columnwise. The electrons in every pixel are shifted to another pixel, by adjusting the voltage barriers of each pixel (Fig. 7.9). Thus, the charge pocket in one column moves in unison and finally reaches the pixel in the bottom row. The bottom row is readout pixel-by-pixel and the charge is shifted to the readout electronics, which produces an electronic signal. This signal is digitized by an *analog-digital converter* (ADC) and the digital signal is used to construct image matrix with bit depth of 8–12.

Similarly, next column charges are shifted to the bottom row that gives another signal. This process is repeated until all the pixels in the detector are readout completely. The readout is faster and it is at the rate of 30 frames per second. The CCD geometry is uniform and distortion-free. It has wide dynamic range with low electronic noise.

Applications of Charge-coupled Devices

Charge-coupled devices produce high quality images and find application in dental radiography, mammography, fluoroscopy, and cineradiography. In dental radiography intensifying screen is coupled with CCD and the field of view (FOV) is too small (25 × 50 mm). The light emitted by the screen is collected by the CCD efficiently. Since the coupling is too good, only little light is wasted.

In digital biopsy mammography, the FOV is higher than the area of the CCD and hence, *fiberoptic taper* is used between the intensifying screen and CCD. The fiberoptic taper acts as a lens and focus the light emitted by the screen on the CCD surface. The input and output surface of the fiberoptic taper is 50 × 50 mm and 25 × 25 mm, respectively. The loss of light is not significant in this system.

In chest radiography, the FOV is larger (35 × 43 cm) than the CCD surface and the amount of light lost is higher (99.7%). The amount of light lost is proportional to the demagnification factor required to couple the input area to the output area. As less number of photons is used to construct an image, a secondary *quantum sink* will occur. This will increase the noise and reduce the image quality. This will also result in higher radiation dose to the patient. Hence, CCD concept is not preferred in chest radiography. Overall, the CCD has the following advantages:
o   No need of scanning
o   Camera geometry is uniform and distortion free
o   Wide dynamic range
o   Low electron noise.

DIGITAL RADIOGRAPHY SYSTEMS

Digital radiography systems consist of large area, flat panel, and solid state detectors with integrated thin film transistor (TFT) readout and having fast access with best image quality. It should have higher spatial resolution, contrast resolution, and dose efficiency. In general, they are available in two configurations, namely:
o   Indirect detection flat panel system
o   Direct detection flat panel system

In indirect systems, the X-rays are converted into light by a phosphor and then light is converted into electric signal. In direct systems, the X-rays are converted directly into an electric signal (Figs. 7.10A and B).

Digital Radiography 137

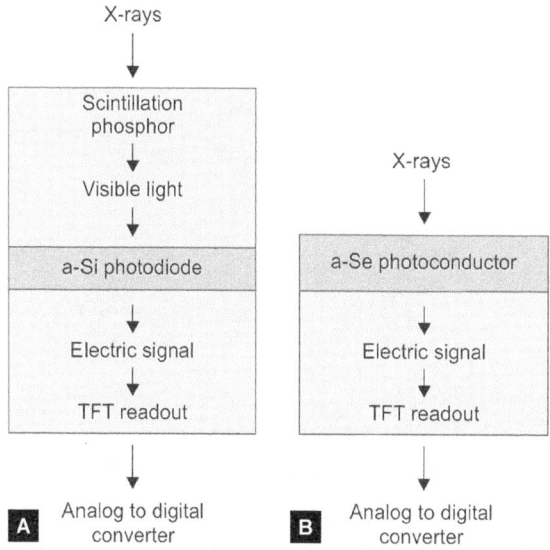

Figs. 7.10A and B: Principle of digital radiography: (A) Indirect and (B) direct detection flat panel systems.
(TFT: Thin film transistor; a-Si: Amorphous silicon; a-Se: Amorphous selenium)

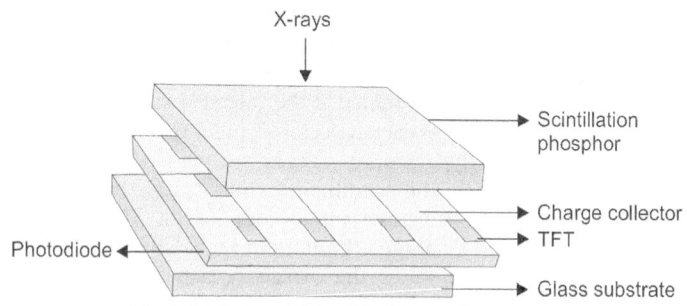

Fig. 7.11: Indirect detection flat panel system.
(TFT: Thin film transistor)

Indirect Detection Flat Panel Systems

Indirect detection flat panel systems consist of a scintillation phosphor, *amorphous silicon (a-Si)*, photodiode, and flat TFT arrays. The scintillation crystal used is *CsI:Tl* or $Gd_2O_2S:Tb$ that converts the incident X-rays into light. It works similar to that of an intensifying screen in a cassette. The detector base is the glass substrate, on to which light sensitive a-Si with a capacitor and TFT is embedded in the form of pixels. The top most component is the scintillation phosphor (Fig. 7.11). Amorphous silicon

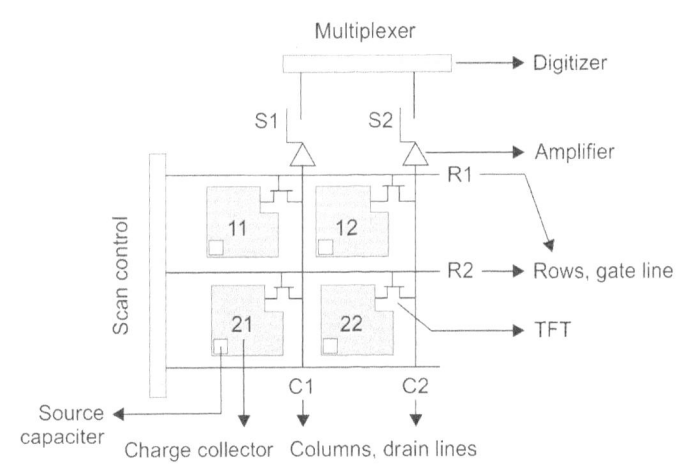

Fig. 7.12: The thin film transistor (TFT) readout process by scan control.

is a fluid that can be painted on a given surface. The entire assembly is put in a protective enclosure with external cable connections. There is no need of fiberoptic guide as in the case of CCD for image demagnification.

The TFT that has three connections, namely; gate, source, and drain, respectively (Fig. 7.12). The source is the capacitor, drain is connected to the readout line (vertical column) and the gate is connected to the horizontal line (rows). TFT is basically an electronic switch that can be made ON and OFF. When negative voltage is applied to the gate, the TFT is said to be OFF and if positive voltage is applied to the gate, it is said to be ON.

Initially, the capacitor of each detector element that stores the charge is earthed, so that all the residual charges are passed on the ground. When exposed to X-rays, the scintillation emits visible light, which in turn exposes the light sensitive photodiode (a-Si). The photodiode releases electrons, so that charge is built up in each detector element that is stored by the capacitor. Later, the charge in each detector element is readout by the electronics as follows.

During the X-ray exposure, negative voltage is applied to the gate and all the transistor switches are in OFF position. The charge accumulated in each detector element is stored in the capacitor. During the readout process, positive voltage is applied to the gate, such a way that one row at a time. Thus, the switches of detector elements in a given row are made ON. This will connect vertical wires C1, C2, to the digitizer through switches S1, and S2, respectively. The multiplexer select the column sequentially (one column at a time) and the charge is amplified and allowed to move to the digitizer. Thus, the gate selects a row and multiplexer selects a column and the charge in each detector element is readout sequentially. Finally, the signal is digitized and stored for image analysis.

Table 7.1: Comparison of CsI:Tl with Gd_2O_2S:Tb phosphor.

S.No.	CsI:Tl	Gd_2O_2S:Tb
1	Z = 55 and K-edge = 33 keV	Z = 64 and K-edge = 50 keV
2	Monoclinic elongated crystal, through light in forward direction	Unstructured crystal as uniform layer, held in a binder
3	Thicker crystal is used to increase DQE	Thinner crystal is used
4	Lesser lateral light spread	Higher lateral light spread
5	Higher spatial resolution	Spatial resolution less
6	Relatively expensive	Cheaper and robust
7	Hygroscopic and quickly degrade	Not applicable

Phosphor Materials

Two types of phosphor materials are commonly used, namely:
- Terbium-doped gadolinium oxysulfide (Gd_2O_2S:Tb)
- Thallium-doped cesium iodide (CsI:Tl).

The Gd_2O_2S:Tb (Z = 64) is an unstructured crystal produced in a uniform layer, held in a binder and it is borrowed from screen-film technology. These systems lose light energy by scatter, accounting lateral light spread. As a result, X-ray photon interaction spreads to adjacent pixels, which reduces the spatial resolution.

CsI:Tl (Z = 55) is obtained from the image intensifier technology. It consists of discrete monoclinic needles of 5–10 μm wide and 600 μm long. These crystals are hygroscopic and quickly degrade, if not completely sealed. Since it pushes the light in the forward direction, light spread is reduced. This facilitates design of thicker phosphor material which increases X-ray photon interaction and quantum efficiency (Table 7.1).

Direct Detection Flat Panel Systems

Direct detection flat panel system uses X-ray photoconductor material like *amorphous selenium* (a-Se, Z = 34), which directly converts X-rays into electrical signal (Fig. 7.13). There is no intermediate material like scintillation phosphor, which converts X-rays into light, as in the case of indirect detector flat panel systems. Since selenium is in amorphous form, large area plates can be made by vapor deposition, which is a cost-effective and reproducible technology. It has good X-ray detection properties and high spatial resolution. Selenium is a photoconductor, and it alters its electrical conductivity, when exposed to X-rays. The altered electrical signal is proportional to the intensity of X-rays.

Initially, 5 kV bias voltage is applied to the surface of the selenium. Later, when it is exposed to X-rays, it emits electrons, which discharge part of the applied voltage. The amount of discharge is proportional to

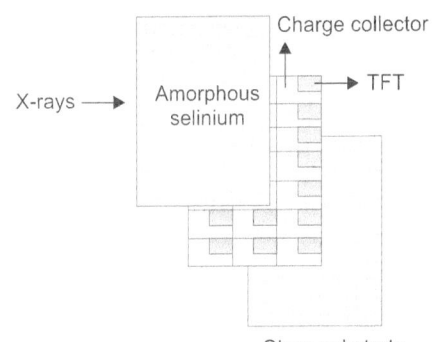

Medical X-ray Film Processing

Fig. 7.13: Direct detection flat panel system.
(TFT: Thin film transistor)

Table 7.2: Comparison of indirect and direct flat panel systems.

S.No.	Indirect flat panel system	Direct flat panel system
1	Silicon phosphor is used: Z = 14	Selenium phosphor is used: Z = 34
2	X-ray is converted into light then electron signal	X-ray is directly converted into electron signal
3	Phosphor is thinner	Phosphor is thicker
4	Causes blur due to light spread	No blurring due to electron travel
5	Fill factor is lower	Fill factor is higher
6	Contrast resolution is poor	Contrast resolution is higher
7	Limited detector size	Large area plate can be made

the radiation intensity, resulting in latent charge image. These charges are stored in the capacitor, and the pattern of charge is readout by scan control lines, similar to that of indirect systems. Finally, the signal is amplified, digitized for image analysis. Selenium is susceptible to humidity and temperature variations, and requires protection from environment. The difference between the indirect and direct flat panel systems are given in Table 7.2. Comparison between computed radiography and digital radiography is given in Table 7.3

Comparison of Detector Systems

Digital radiography systems should have high signal-noise ratio and provide connectivity to DICOM, hospital information system (HIS), and radiological information system (RIS). The probability of photon interaction with detector material is given by the detective quantum efficiency and it is higher for gadolinium oxysulfide. This can be increased by increasing the detector thickness and materials having

Digital Radiography

Table 7.3: Comparison of computed radiography and digital radiography systems.

S.No.	Computed radiography	Digital radiography
1	*Versatility:* Single cassette is used both for table and stand buchy	Require two separate detectors for table and stand buchy
2	*Flexibility:* Oblique view and bed side X-ray is possible	Do not have the same flexibility
3	Single CR system can support multiple X-ray units	Each room requires independent DR system
4	No need for X-ray equipment modification	X-ray equipment need replacement
5	DQE is about 30%	DQE is about 65%
6	Throughput is lower	Throughput is higher
7	Available at lower cost	Relatively expensive

high attenuation coefficient. Both direct and indirect detector system have wide dynamic range, compared to screen-film system. However, in practice, this wide range is restrictively used, because low exposure gives noisy image and high exposure increases patient dose.

The light collection efficiency of each detector element depends on the fractional area that is sensitive to light, which is defined by the *fill factor* as follows:

Fill factor = Light sensitive area/area of detector element

In DR, detector is occupied by conductors, capacitors and TFT, and only partial area of the detector is sensitive to X-rays (Fig. 7.14A). Hence,

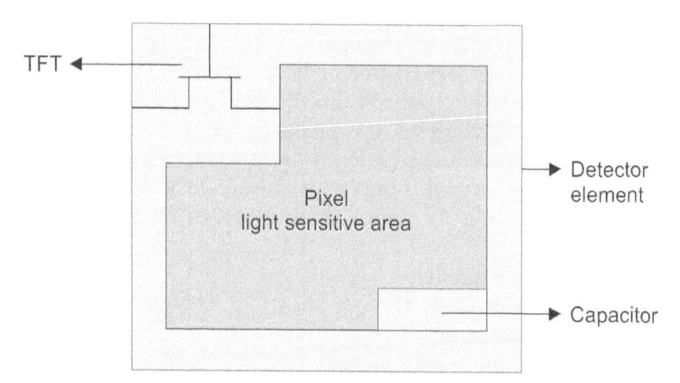

Fig. 7.14A: Fill factor is the ratio of the light sensitive area to detector element area.
(TFT: Thin film transistor)

142 Medical X-ray Film Processing

```
     Light sensitive area          Detector element


          High                        Medium                     Low
```

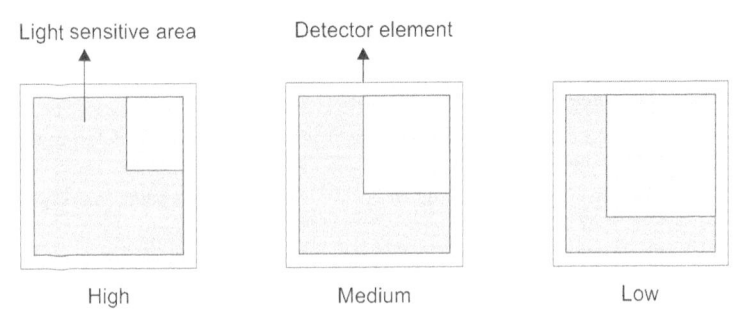

Fig. 7.14B: Fill factor, as the light sensitive area decreases the fill factor also decreases.

the fill factor is always less than 100% and this will vary depending upon the detector system. The fill factor is higher for direct a-Se system, compared to indirect DR systems.

Small detector element gives higher spatial resolution, but reduces the fill factor. As the light sensitive area decreases, fill factor also decreases (Fig. 7.14B). Low fill factor reduces the signal-noise ratio, resulting in poor contrast resolution. Hence, there is tradeoff between spatial resolution and contrast resolution for a given detector. For better understanding the reader, a comparison or differences between the screen-film and digital radiography system is highlighted in Table 7.4.

Portable Flat Panel Cassette

Nowadays, mobile DR X-ray machines are used with portable flat panel cassettes, which can be inserted in a standard buchy tray cabinet or a CR system. Initially, these cassettes are wired to the X-ray generator, for image acquisition. Of late, wireless detectors with full field automatic exposure detection (AED) technology is available (Fig. 7.15). Cassettes are made available with active area of 10"x 12"-11" x 17", pixel area of 2816 x 2816 and pixel pitch of 154 µm. It provides large area coverage and unrestricted time windows. It is precalibrated and user friendly and known as *direct digital*. These cassettes are provided with handle with drop protection and smooth nonporous surface. It is light weight and has durability and long life time. These cassettes have the following advantages:

○ Consistent image quality
○ Reduced radiation dose
○ Faster image formation
○ Same size as a film or a CR cassette
○ DICOM complaint
○ Low noise
○ High MTF

Digital Radiography

Table 7.4: Comparison of screen-film with digital radiography system.

S.No.	Screen-Film radiography	Digital Radiography (CR/DR)
1	X-ray film with cassette is used	Photostimulable phosphor (PSP) as imaging plate is used in CR. Flat panels are used in DR
2	Used with intensifying screens, emits either blue or green light	No need for intensifying screens, emits blue-green and ultraviolet
3	Speed is defined for a given screen-film combination and has limitation	No such limitation
4	Dark room with processing chemicals (developer and fixer) are required	No darkroom and chemicals are required. Instead CR reader is used. Single reader can support multiple X-ray units
5	Film contains 7–26 g of silver per kg, and involves silver recovery	No such requirements
6	Film gives analog image	CR/DR gives digital image
7	Electronic storage not possible, only film can be scanned and stored	Electronic storage and retrieval of image is possible
8	Image capture, storage and display are performed by screen-film system	Image capture, storage and display are independent
9	Film cannot be reused	Can be reused, with reproducible results
10	Work flow is similar and patient throughput is same	Work flow is similar and patient throughput is same
11	No provision for post processing: retake rate is higher	Provision for post processing and manipulation of data (edge enhancement). Retake rate is lower
12	Technologist has limitation to select his exposure settings (kV, mAs)	Technologist has more freedom to select his own exposure technique (kV, mAs)
13	Available sizes: 7"×7", 8" × 10", 10" × 12", 14" × 14" and 14" × 17"	Available sizes: 8" × 10", 10" × 12", 14" × 14" and 14" × 17"
14	X-ray film latitude is narrow and has small dynamic range: 1:1000	Has wider dynamic range (1:10,000) and has wider latitude, able to show low contrast differences
15	Amount of radiation required to produce a good image is fixed: 5 µGy for 200 speed film	It can accept 100 times either low or higher radiation exposure
16	Detective quantum efficiency: 15%	Detective quantum efficiency: 25% for CR and 50% for DR
17	Spatial resolution is 8–12 lp/mm	3.5-5.5 lp/mm
18	kV controls the contrast and mA controls the optical density	Not valid here. CR image contrast is constant, irrespective of exposure techniques

Contd...

Medical X-ray Film Processing

Contd...

S.No.	Screen-Film radiography	Digital Radiography (CR/DR)
19	Source of noises are from quantum mottle and screen-film	Source of noises are from scatter radiation, drive mechanism, laser and computer devices
20	Image quality depends on contrast, spatial resolution, sharpness, noise and geometric factors	Depends on spatial resolution, noise, detective quantum efficiency of the phosphor
21	Film is relatively slow, involves higher patient dose	Faster, images can be produced with lower patient dose
22	Less expensive initially, but costlier on long run, with lower operation efficiency	Expensive at the initial phase, cheaper on long run with higher operational efficiency
23	Not possible	Computer network permits image sharing and exchange of information. On line imaging is possible
24	Not possible	Since images are in DICOM format, use of PACS and Tele radiology is possible.
25	Photodiode is used to detect detector dose, automatic exposure control (AEC) is employed.	Difficult to access detector dose, require elaborate quality assurance.

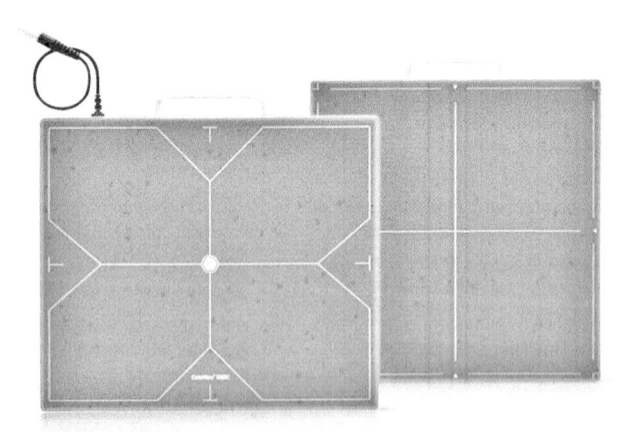

Fig. 7.15: A commercial portable flat panel detector.
(*Courtesy*: M/s Careray digital Medical, Technologies, China)

- High DQE
- Easy patient positioning
- Increased workflow
- Easy to clean and disinfect

- Excellent contrast detail
- Exam dependent
- Consistent image quality.

They basically use either CsI:Tl or Gd_2O_2S:Tb(GOS) crystals for making the detector. CsI crystals are grown in a controlled condition and deposited directly on flat panels and sealed with a hermetic packing. It is made with water resistant Al-alloy or Magnesium alloy frame, combined with carbon fiber and impact absorbing rubber edging. The CsI gives excellent image quality, fast image availability with significant dose reduction. On the other hand, GOS detectors are cost-effective with excellent image quality.

It can transfer image data within few seconds with high transmission rate. It is also provided with battery support (up to 8 hrs), which can offer more than 1000 shots with 10s interval between shots. These images can be stored, and captured image is validated immediately. Option of retrieving old images stored previously is also available.

Cassette holder is also available for easy positioning. These holders can be rotated up to 180/360 degree, or any angle from the floor level to 180 cm. They do have the provision to insert DR cassette with grid. It has wide application; general radiography, pediatric radiography, extremities and special examinations. It can also be effectively used in NICU, OT and emergency imaging.

8
Digital Radiography; Image Quality, Viewing, and Recording

IMAGE QUALITY

Digital radiography offers on line imaging and the image is read out from the receptor quickly. There is no need to remove the receptor, which increases patient throughput. The images can be transmitted electronically and identical copy of the image can be made. Use of computer for image archiving, and post adjustment of contrast is also possible. This will result in improved interpretation and improved diagnosis. The various factors that influence the image quality are as follows:
- Spatial resolution
- Contrast resolution
- Noise
- Detective quantum efficiency.

The above parameters have been used to analyze screen-film radiography images. In the same way, digital image can also be analyzed. This will enable us to understand not only the image characteristics, but also to compare them with conventional radiography images.

Spatial Resolution

The spatial resolution is the ability to resolve a small high-contrast object and record its image. It is generally designed by the size of the object. The spatial resolution of our human eye is 200 μm. This means that the smallest object size that one can see is 200 μm. Generally, black on light background have higher contrast, while gray shades have lesser contrast. If the object is made up of gray shades, contrast decreases, the eye cannot see 200 μm sizes object and requires higher object size. Higher is the contrast, lesser the object size to be seen.

However, spatial resolution is described in terms of spatial frequency in medical imaging, not by the size of the object. Usually, spatial frequency refers line pairs (lp), that is a black line on a white background. One lp consists of a line and an interspace (Fig. 8.1). It is expressed as line pair per millimeter (lp/mm).

The spatial resolution of screen-film radiography is about 8 lp/mm, whereas, it is 4 lp/mm for digital radiography (DR). This is the maximum limitation in DR, due to its pixel size. However, spatial frequency and object size are interlinked. If the spatial frequency is 4 lp/mm, one can see 8 objects in 1 mm, including the interface. Then, the size of the object is 1/8 mm = 0.125.

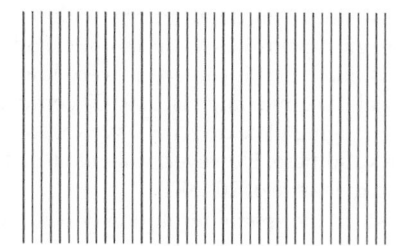

Fig. 8.1: Line pair.

Sampling Frequency

In the case of digital system, sampling frequency determines the spatial resolution. Sampling frequency is the number of samples per mm, which is determined by the matrix size. A matrix size of 100 x 100 covering an anatomical length of 10 mm, gives 100 samples in 10 mm or 10 samples in per mm. This means that each pixel will contribute one sample. If the matrix size is doubled, pixel size reduces to half, and the sampling frequency is doubled. The sampling frequency is related to the spatial resolution as follows:

Spatial resolution = ½ x sample frequency or pixel spacing

If the sampling frequency is 10 per mm, then the spatial resolution is 5 lp/mm. Such a system can resolve 5 line pairs of black and white. The maximum resolution that can be obtained in an imaging system is called *Nyquist frequency*.

Nyquist Frequency

Consider a detector of pixel width d mm, from center to center. If two pixels (2d) covers a full cycle of a signal (Both maxima and minima), then the period is 2d mm. The spatial frequency = 1/period = 1/2d, which is called Nyquist frequency. This gives the upper limit to detect images, in terms of spatial frequency. If the signal frequency is greater, the detector will not record the signal. The signal is said to be aliased and the event is called aliasing. This may lead to improper reconstruction of image from the original. Aliasing may cause wraparound images, called *aliasing artifacts*. Thus, Nyquist frequency sets upper limitation to the spatial resolution.

Digital Radiography Resolution

Digital radiography employs a matrix size of 2000 x 2500 over an anatomical dimension of 350 x 430 mm, and the sampling frequency is about 6 per mm. The limiting spatial resolution is ½ x 6 = 3 lp/mm. The above is a high resolution (HR) plate and is digitized to 10 bits. Standard resolution (ST) plates are available with 1760 x 2140 matrix size, and digitized to 10 bits. Chest radiography employs a matrix size of 3584 x 4096. These are 12 bit depth matrix with a resolution of 5–10 pixels per mm. Imaging plate has wide latitude and dynamic range. Its dynamic range is linear and it can accept very low to high radiation exposures. The actual dynamic range is 1:10,000 compared to 1:1000 for screen-film system. Imaging plate does not have speed limitation and the concept is no more valid here. However, it is rated that the speed of an imaging plate lies in the range of 20–2000.

In flat panel system, the spatial resolution depends on pixel spacing in the detector. Nyquist frequency decides the limiting spatial resolution. The MTF of the direct flat panel system is high enough to view minute diagnostic details. The factors that influences the spatial resolution are:
- Focal spot size
- Magnification
- Phantom scattering
- Patient motion
- Aperture size
- Spatial sampling interval between measurement and lateral scattering effects of X-rays.

The top four factors are extrinsic and the last two are intrinsic in nature.

Fluoroscopy Resolution

Digital fluoroscopy uses a matrix size of about 1000 x 1000. If it views a FOV of 250 mm, then there will be 4 samples per mm. The corresponding spatial resolution is ½ x 4 = 2 lp/mm. The above resolution can be improved by the reduction of FOV. In the case of a flat panel system, the sampling frequency is fixed. Hence, its resolution is independent of FOV. The achievable resolution in digital mammography is 10 lp/mm.

CT Scan Resolution

Digital CT scan employs 512 x 512 matrix sixe. In head scan imaging, it covers 250 mm of anatomical length and the sampling frequency is about 1 lp/mm. In abdomen scan, it covers over 350 mm of anatomy, and the sampling frequency is 1.4 per mm. The achievable resolution is about 0.7 lp/mm.

Thus, CT resolution is much lower than the screen-film radiography (8 lp/mm) and digital radiography (3 lp/mm).To improve the resolution in CT scan, large matrix size or small focal spot can be used. Large matrix size does not alter resolution much, due to inbuilt focal spot and detector blur. High resolution (HR) CT with small FOV can improve CT axial resolution. Employing small focus or smaller detector can also improve CT resolution. Detector width decides the resolution in longitudinal direction.

Modular Transfer Function

The modular transfer function (MTF) is the ratio of output to input modulation as a function of spatial frequency. An ideal image is one

Digital Radiography; Image Quality, Viewing, and Recording 149

which produces an image that appears exactly as the object; in that case the MTF is unity. In clinical practice, there is no such ideal imaging system; the MTF is always < 1. The MTF and the spatial frequency can be plotted in a graph (Fig. 6.4, Chapter 6).

If the spatial frequency is lesser, the MTF is higher and the system will have good visibility with added features. On the other hand, higher spatial frequency does have lower MTF and reproduction of image is difficult. It will have poor visibility with less features. In other words, at low spatial frequency, the image contrast is preserved. At high spatial frequency the image contrast is low.

Generally, an imaging system has multiple components. The MTF of a given system is the product of MTF of the individual subsystems. MTF analysis may be helpful to understand imaging system performance.

Contrast Resolution

The contrast resolution is the ability to differentiate many shades of gray from black to white. Digital radiography has better contrast resolution compared to screen-film radiography. It is described by the parameter; grayscale or dynamic range.

Dynamic range of an imaging system is the number of gray shade that it can reproduce. In screen-film radiography, the optical density range is 0–3, which represents a dynamic range of 1,000. However, one can visualize only 30 shades of gray, due to limitation of human eye.

On the other hand, the DR, dynamic range is 14 bit capacity corresponding to 2^{14} = 16,384 shades of gray. Here, the dynamic range is described by the pixel size and bit capacity. The dynamic range of computed tomography (CT) and magnetic resonance imaging (MRI) is of the order of 2^{12}, whereas, it is 2^{16} for mammography. However, human eye cannot visualize all the grayscales. To overcome this, postprocessing of the image is done with window width and window level. This will enable us to expand any part of the 16,384 grayscales into white to black. Thus, DR offers about 4–5 times more response than screen-film radiography, for a given exposure technique. One can also visualize all the grayscales by image postprocessing process. This is clinically beneficial, especially in soft tissue imaging.

The contrast resolution is limited by noise or signal to noise ratio (SNR). The signal is the amount of X-rays that forms the anatomy. This depends on the difference between the X-rays transmitted to the detector and the X-rays absorbed in the human body.

Noise

Noise limits the ability to view a lesion or pathology in an digital image. A noisy image may appear as grainy or mottled. Noise in the digital image is due to scatter radiation and detector system. Noise in the image quality depends on the quantum efficiency of the phosphor, charge collection by the capacitor and noise free read out of the stored signal. The indirect detector system uses light that undergoes scatter, resulting in reduction of signal-to-noise ratio. One should always look for high SNR, to preserve contrast resolution. This will satisfy ALARA principle of radiation safety.

The digital radiography offers better low contrast resolution than screen-film. However, they suffer from inferior spatial resolution. The noise in the PSP imaging plate arises from the following ways:
- Quantum noise
- Light photon noise
- Fixed noise.

An acceptable quantum noise is obtained up to 100 µGy, which is ensured in the imaging plate design. This is not true at higher doses, beyond 100 µGy. Quantum noise can be reduced by reducing the thickness of the protective layer of the phosphor. The light photon noise arises from the photo multiplier tube (PMT). It is due to fluctuations of photo electrons at the PMT. Hence, PMT should have high photoelectric conversion efficiency. Fixed noise arises in the form of structural, imaging plate, laser, analog circuit and quantization noises. Structural noise dominates over others, and it can be reduced by having reduced grain size. In the flat panel system, noise arises from the following:
- Quantum efficiency of the phosphor
- Capacitor charge collection
- Readout.

In the indirect flat panel, X-rays is converted into light and later as electron charge signal. The light photon undergoes scatter before reaching the TFT and reduces SNR. However, this is avoided in the direct flat panel system.

Digital fluoroscopy exposure techniques are similar to image intensifier tube system. Frame averaging is the concept used here to reduce noise. The noise in the digital CT is 3 HU, which is due to random fluctuations in attenuation coefficient. The primary cause of noise depends on number of X-ray photons that makes the image. This is in turn depends on mA and tube voltage. The noise is inversely proportional to $mAs^{0.5}$. Increasing the kV may reduce CT noise. Use of filters will increase noise, but soft tissue filter reduce noise with increase of spatial resolution.

Detective Quantum Efficiency

Radiological image quality is evaluated by resolution, modular transfer function, contrast, and mottle, etc, over the years. But, they are not adequate to evaluate the performance of an imaging system. Basically, an imaging system is made up of several subcomponents.

Digital Radiography; Image Quality, Viewing, and Recording

The signal-to-noise ratio (SNR) is not the same at various stages of the subcomponents. X-rays are polyenergetic in nature, and effective energy is always used. Hence, the X-ray spectrum incident on the detector is an effective quantum efficiency type. In the case of digital setup, image can be processed unlimitedly to improve image quality. This may lead to increased noise in the image, which will alter the output signal-to-noise ratio (output SNR). Hence, the output SNR is different from the input signal-noise ratio (input SNR).

Hence, there is need for a single parameter, to address the above issues. The detective quantum efficiency (DQE) is such a parameter, which comprehensively evaluate the performance of an imaging system. It replaces the above said terms; resolution, MTF, contrast, and mottle as well as the subcomponents of an imaging system. The DQE is expressed in terms of ratio of the SNR:

$$DQE = \frac{Output\ SNR^2}{Input\ SNR^2}$$

It describes the imaging system's accuracy of response towards radiation. The DQE of film is maximum over the optical density of 1 and 2. Therefore, film processing is very much critical to achieve the above density. In screen-film system, to improve resolution thin screen phosphor is suggested. This will increase the noise, resulting in low output SNR and reduces the DQE. Hence, optimal balance is required between resolution and noise. The screen-film system is capable of detecting even a small anatomy of the order of 130 µm.

In fluoroscopy, usually the noise levels are higher, since less number of photons is making the image. The DQE relates the input screen absorption efficiency and its X-ray–to-light conversion efficiency to obtain the SNR figure. The dynamic range is decided by the electronic noise and video camera. The DQE measurement takes into account the number of photons reaching the input window, absorbed by the input screen and photons forming the image. DQE values for fluoroscopy ranges from 50–70%.

Digital Radiography (CR/DR)

In computed radiography, the DQE evaluates the sensitivity and image quality. It serves as an index and addresses resolution, contrast and mottle. The comparison of DQE for screen-film system with that of CR is given in Figure 8.2. The CR system DQE is better than the screen-film at spatial frequency, where the X-ray exposure levels are 10–25 µGy (<2 lp/mm). At higher special frequency (>2 lp/mm), it falls rapidly, due to noise from various sources. The limiting spatial resolution of the CR system is 5lp/mm, whereas it is 15 lp/mm, for screen-film system.

In the case flat panel system, quantum efficiency is much more important. The probability of photon interaction with the detector plays

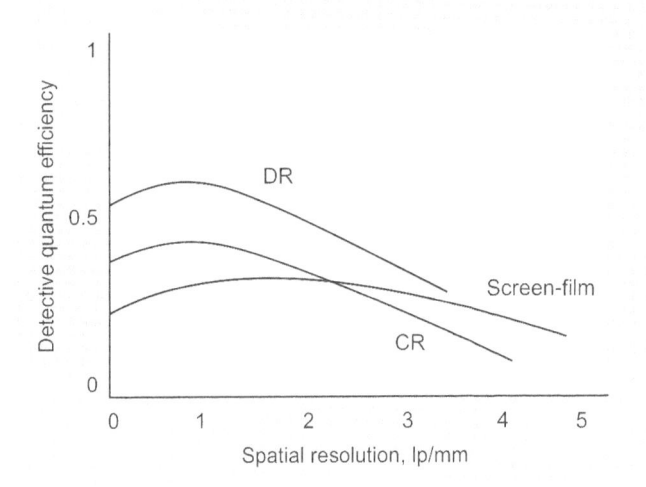

Fig. 8.2: Variation of DQE against Spatial resolution, for DR, Screen-film and CR system.

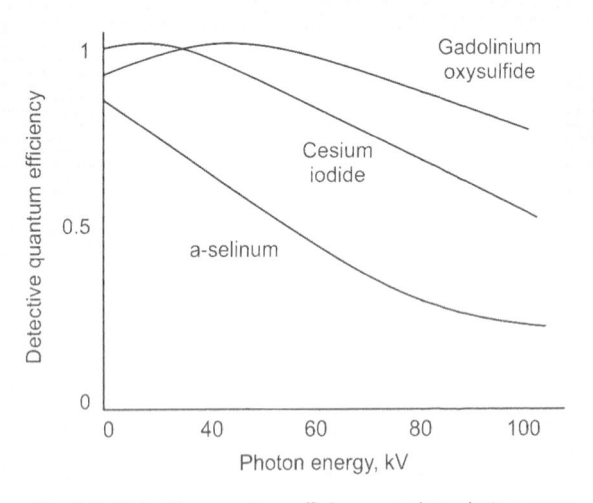

Fig. 8.3: Detective quantum efficiency against photo energy.

an vital role here. It depends on the linear attenuation coefficient (μ) and thickness of detector material and photon energy. The DQE is increased by increasing the quantum efficiency. That means, DQE is increased by increasing the detector thickness and having high μ. The DQE is higher for gadolinium oxysulfide over the photon energy of 40–100 kV (Fig. 8.3).

The drop in DQE is greater at higher energy, greater for selenium. Overall, DQE is higher at low photon energy and it decreases with increase of photon energy, after the K-edge. The DQE of a CR and DR system is about 25% and 50% respectively, whereas it is 15% for screen-film system.

DQE differs between indirect and direct flat panel system. The various factors that affect the DQE are:
○ Noise
○ Readout
○ Dynamic range
○ Quantum efficiency.

In indirect system, the X-ray interaction depth at the scintillator decides the brightness and lateral spread, leading to noise. This is totally absent in the direct flat panel system, especially at high spatial frequency. In the direct flat panel, the number electrons produced and lateral spread are independent of depth.

The indirect detector system suffers due to light scattering, and there is tradeoff between X-ray absorption and MTF. Thinner scintillation crystal gives high MTF, but reduces X-ray absorption. Thicker crystal increases the X-ray absorption, but reduces the MTF, due to increase of light scatter. In the case of direct detector system, the thickness can be increased, so that X-ray absorption can be increased without loss of MTF.

The selenium detector has high quantum efficiency and dynamic range, compared to others. It does not require a read out facility. It is not influenced by light scatter and detector thickness. The detector receives the X-ray without much loss. Hence, it is superior than other detectors in terms of noise reduction and image quality. The DQE of selenium decreases both in terms of higher spatial resolution and higher photon energy. It scores well in terms of spatial resolution over gadolinium detector. But gadolinium scores over selenium in terms of photon energy. However, selenium is susceptible to humidity and temperature, compared to other detectors. Hence, it should be protected from environmental factors.

DQE is the best parameter to evaluate image quality and performance of an imaging system. It addresses both special resolution and noise of the system in a combined way. It provides measure of SNR for various subcomponents of the imaging system. DQE can be measured by using an Am-241 source, which is equivalent to 120 kV X-rays. To measure the output, *photometer* with time constant is used. The integration time should match the human eye. DQE is dose dependent and always stated with radiation dose. It varies with kV and radiation exposure. DQE influences the patient dose and it depends on the input SNR. Higher is the DQE, better the image quality. The expected DQE is about 100, that means the input and output SNR should be the same. No such imaging system is available as on date, and DQE is always less than 100%, due to inefficiency in incident X-ray detection, and internal source of noise.

DIGITAL IMAGE VIEWING

In screen-film radiography, all images are made in X-ray film, as hard copy. However, in DR, the image is in a display monitor, pre- and post-processed and then printed in a special film by a *dry/laser printer*. The detail and design of the printer is explained in the latter paragraphs. This is the final hard copy, which is viewed with the help of view box. They are generally known as *medical imaging workstations*. A typical workstation consists of following:
- Computer
- Operating system software
- Display processing software
- Display controller
- Display device.

The medical imaging image display devices are of *three type*, namely:
- Cathode-ray tube (CRT)
- Active matrix liquid crystal display (AMLCD)
- Flat panel display.

Computer

The computer includes a central processing unit (CPU), mathematical computation modules, input/output (I/O) controllers, and network communication hardware. It also has keyboard, mouse, trackball or wheel, joystick, and barcode scanner. Storage or recording devices such as hard disk, digital video disk (DVD), compact disk (CD) and output devices such as display monitors, printers, and speakers are also incorporated. There are also supporting hardware and software components. The display controller hardware converts digital information into analog or digital signal, suitable to the display device. Software module allows programs to assess the controller hardware. The user application program accesses image data and sends it to the display controller in a suitable format. The special feature of medical imaging computers is that it uses special display software, high resolution display devices, and high performance display controller devices. The above is the basic difference from the general computer.

Operating System Software

Operating system (OS) software is required to perform the function of hard disk, CPU, I/O devices and printer. It is a low level program that controls the resources of the computer. It supports network communication, security, display, and file management and execution of application programs. OS also provides time sharing, so that multiple programs are processed simultaneously. It also monitors keyboard, mouse, network, and other devices. Thus, OS creates an operating environment for the user and for application programs. The software in medical devices is UNIX, LINUX, Macintosh, and Microsoft windows systems.

Digital Radiography; Image Quality, Viewing, and Recording 155

Display Processing Software

Digital image consists of array of digital grayscale values. The display device should transform the grayscale values in to luminance values. The values used by different modalities like CT and DR is different. In general, images are stored initially with specific values, and converted into analog or digital voltages for presentation on a display device. In DR, the stored images are converted to digital driving levels (DDLs), before obtaining analog or digital images with the help of OS. In addition, coloring the image is also done in display processing.

Display Controller

The display controller is nothing but video card or graphic card. It is a combination of hardware and software to transform DDLs to appropriate signals for display device. Most of the display devices accept only analog video signals. In that case, the controller performs digital-analog (D-A) conversion. In flat panel devices, the controller sends the digital signal to display device, and the device converts this to a suitable signal to control luminance.

Display Device

The display device generates a visible image from analog video signals. In addition, it has internal software to respond to the controller commands. A single workstation can have multiple display devices, e.g. 1–2. Either cathode-ray tube (CRT) or flat panels are used as the display device.

Cathode-ray Tube

The cathode ray tube consists of the following components (Fig. 8.4):
- An electron gun
- Control grid (G_1)

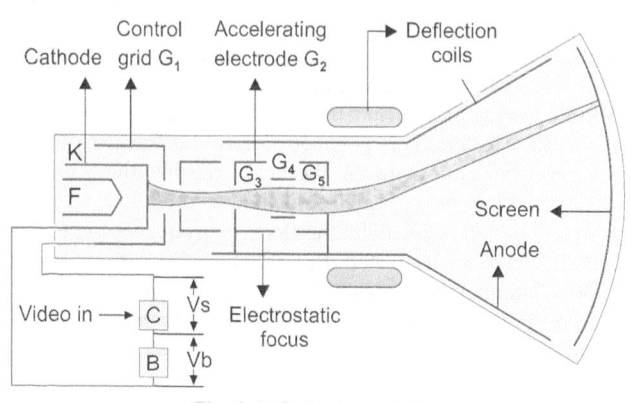

Fig. 8.4: Cathode-ray tube.

- Accelerating electrode (G_2)
- Electrostatic focus (G_3, G_4, G_5)
- Deflection coils
- Anode
- Fluorescent screen
- A glass envelope.

There are two set of deflection coils, namely vertical and horizontal, which are applied saw tooth potential of the order of 140 kHz. The values of the horizontal and vertical control voltage determine the beam position. Horizontal deflection coils produce vertical magnetic field, so that the electron beam is swept from left to right, while line scanning. The vertical deflection coils move the beam downward, after each frame is completed, and bring back the beam to the starting point.

The electron gun produces electrons by thermionic emission, which travel toward the anode and fluorescent screen. The electrons are drawn through G1 (1,000 V) and then G2 (+25 kV). The beam comes to focus at G2 and then diverges. The anode is made up of aluminum layer with reflection yoke at the backside. The intensity of the electron beam is modulated by the control grid. The electron beam is focused on the fluorescent screen with the help of electrostatic focus. The focused electron beam on the phosphor is of the order of 0.1–0.2 mm diameter. The video signal modulates the electron beam and a visible image is formed at the fluorescent screen.

The fluorescent screen consists of a phosphor with linear crystals. It is supported by a thin layer of aluminum at the back side. The aluminum allows only electrons, but reflects light coming from the phosphor. When the electrons interact with the phosphor, light is produced, which gives the final image. The light distribution character on the screen follows *Gaussian function* and *Lambertian distribution*. The rate at which the visible light is emitted is called luminescence. These monitors can produce luminescence of up to 500 cd/m^2.

In a monochromatic CRT device, the electron movement on the fluorescent screen follows *raster pattern*. That is, it travels from left to right, called an *active trace*. Then the electron beam is turned off, and moves from right to left. This is called horizontal trace. After series of such active and horizontal traces, the beam reaches the bottom of the screen. The whole process completes one television field.

To start second television field, the electron beam goes to the top of the screen and the process is repeated. But, this time the active trace is done between the adjacent active traces of the first television field. This is called *interlace*. Two interlaced television fields form a single television frame. Usually, a frame rate of 25/30 is used in medical digital monitors. In India, since the power supply has 50 Hz frequency, it gives 50 television fields and 25 television frames per second. In home television, 16 frame/s is used.

Digital Radiography; Image Quality, Viewing, and Recording

In color CRT, 3 electron guns are used. Screen phosphor is illuminated by the electron beams and gives red, green and blue light. The type of screen phosphor used will determine the color. However, it is difficult to get correct electron focusing. Hence, *shadow mask* or *aperture grill* is used, to overcome the above.

Shadow mask contains a matrix of round aperture in front of the screen pixel. This masks the electron beam more sharper, without color blurring. However, it also prevents electron beams to reach the phosphor, resulting in reduced light intensity. Aperture grill tube consists of a mask made up of vertical wires, which is kept behind the screen. Each pixel is made by 3 vertical wires, for each red, blue and green color, respectively. It enhances the display with better contrast. However, it increases veiling glare, as pixels/line increases.

Active Matrix Liquid Crystal Display

The active matrix liquid crystal display (AMLCD) consists of liquid crystal. It has ordered molecular structure with properties of fluid viscosity. Basically, the liquid crystal materials are linear organic molecules. When they are charged electrically, they can form molecular dipole (Fig. 8.5). This can be done with the help of external electrical field.

The AMLCD is arranged pixel-by-pixel and each pixel is illuminated by white back light. This light illumination is either blocked or transmitted by the orientation of the liquid crystals. Each pixel consists of light polarizing filter and film, which controls the intensity and color of light. Generally, color AMLCD uses red-green-blue filters. However, medical flat panel systems use monochrome (single color) AMLCDs. Each pixel is controlled by a thin film transistor (TFT).

Generally, medical flat panel digital display systems are classified by number of pixels in the AMLCD, e.g. one mega pixel (MP) display

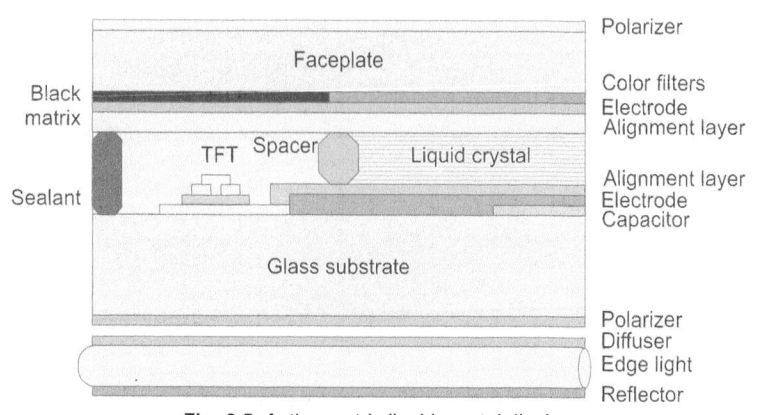

Fig. 8.5: Active matrix liquid crystal display.

monitor may have 1000 × 1000 pixels. On the other hand, 2 MP, 3 MP, and 5 MP will have 1200 × 1800, 1500 × 200, and 2000 × 2500 pixels, respectively. Display monitor efficiency is defined by aperture ratio. It is the part of the pixel area that is available for light transmission. Generally, aperture ratio ranges from 50% to 80%. AMLCDs are designed with flat surface with better grayscale definition and better contrast resolution. This is the advantage of AMLCD over CRT monitors that have curved surface.

Flat Panel Monitor

The purpose of the monitor is to convert the electronic signal into visual display. Earlier CRT was used and slowly replaced by flat monitor systems. They basically use liquid crystals or plasma to give better images. The flat panel systems are divided into following category:
- Liquid crystal display (LCD)
- Plasma display panel (PDP)
- Light emitting diode (LED).

The LCD monitor screens consist of a back light and liquid crystal. Back light is a series of light tubes placed behind the screen. They are similar to fluorescent lamps, but smaller in size. LCD screen does not emit light by itself it acts only as filter to block the light on per pixel basis. The fluorescent lamps that are used are called *cold-cathode fluorescent lamps* (CCFL). The liquid crystal system acts as a filter and either block or permits light transmission.

The liquid crystals are in the form of semi liquid. It is a thin nematic crystal, similar to rod shaped and exists in an unorganized state. The LCD has several layers as shown in Figure 8.6. The liquid crystal is the main component and it is sandwiched between polarized films/filter.

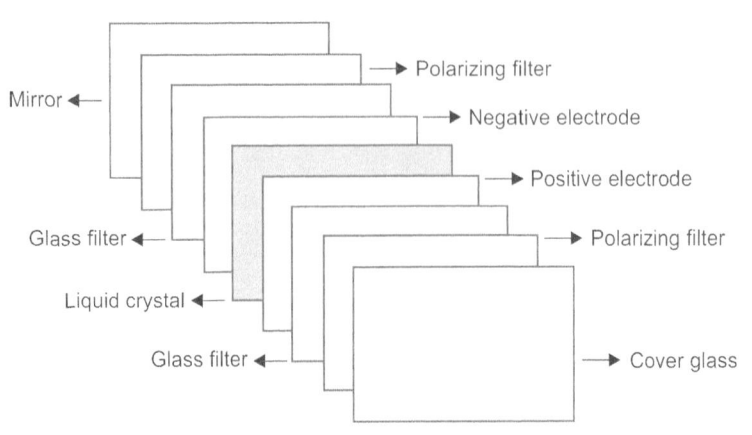

Fig. 8.6: Flat panel display system: Liquid crystal display (LCD) and its components.

The crystal has electrodes both in front and back. The liquid crystal exists initially in an unorganized state. When an electric current is passed, the crystal undergoes a twist. In addition, it has a mirror, glass filter and cover glass. The polarizing filter is rod shaped and both filters are kept at 90°. That is, if one filter is in vertical and other one is in horizontal orientation. TFT panel is there behind the liquid crystal and each pixel has one TFT. The TFT controls the current to each pixel. When there is no electric current, the light emission is blocked by the polarizing filter. Once the TFT supply electric current, the crystal undergo a twist and permits the light to transmit. Thus, switching ON and OFF of the TFT, make the electric current either absent or present in the liquid crystal. Therefore, the crystal undergoes no twist or twist; other words either block or permit light transmission forward. The degree of twist depends on the supply of electric current by TFT. Thus, the TFT controls the electric current, crystal twist and light intensity.

In plasma display panel, thin layer of pixel is used, and each pixel is made of 3 neon and xenon gas filled cells. Each cell is coated with different phosphor layer, that will produce red, green and blue light. The plasma layer is sandwiched between dielectric layer. If current is passed through the dielectric layer, it passes through the pixels, and ionizes the gas. As a result, electrons are liberated, which release ultraviolet light (UV). The UV light stimulates the phosphor to emit light. The color of the light emission depends upon the phosphor for which it is coded. The current through the pixel is modulated by the electrodes at a high rate (> 1000 time/s). Thus, the emitted light intensity is controlled. Plasma monitors are capable of producing billions of color shades. Though the motion blur is less in the system, they suffer from image retention. Hence, this type of monitor is no longer available in the market.

The light emitting diode monitor is similar to that of LCD monitor. The only difference is the back light. It uses light emitting diodes as back light, instead of CCFL. The LED is more energy efficient and smaller than CCFL. This enabled to make smaller TV monitors. There is no much improvement in picture quality between LCD and LED.

Pre- and Postprocessing

One of the principal advantages of digital image is pre- and postprocessing. This will alter the image appearance with better contrast. Preprocessing includes the following:
○ Defective pixel interpolation
○ Image lag
○ Noise correction.

Pixel interpolation addresses defective pixel. If any one of the pixels is defective, the response of adjacent pixels is interpolated and the same is assigned to the defective pixel.

Secondly image lag; in this the electronic latent image is not made visible completely. This may arise when we switch over from one procedure to another, e.g. digital subtraction angiography (DSA) to fluoroscopy. This can be overcome by application of offset voltage.

Thirdly noise correction; any voltage variation leads to line noise, resulting in image artifacts. All the above preprocessing is done automatically in the system before the image display.

Postprocessing is done after the image display. It is performed with the help of technologists or radiologists. The purpose of postprocessing is to optimize the image appearance, to detect pathology. The various post-processing steps include the following:
- Annotation
- Window width and window level
- Magnification
- Image flip
- Image inversion
- Subtraction
- Pixel shift
- Region of interest
- Edge enhancement
- Smoothening equalization.

Annotation is labeling the image by adding text. This contains patient information, examination, site, reference, etc. Text can be added to the image to identify regions of interest. Adjusting window width and window level, one can easily see all shades of gray up to 16,000. For example, 16-bit image may have 65,536 gray shades, which can be seen fully with window width and window level adjustments. This is the most important advantage of digital image. Magnification helps to see smallest detail of the image. This will improve visualization and spatial resolution. A small electronic magnifying lens is provided in the system, to see fine details. The image flip is the process in which the image is flipped either horizontally or vertically. This will standardize the image viewing order, so that proper orientation of image is obtained for further interpretation. Generally, bone appears as white and soft tissue as black. In image inversion, it can be reversed. That is, bone appears as black and soft tissue as white. In addition, image can be changed from negative to positive or vice-versa. This will help to identify pathology more visible.

The purpose of image subtraction is to improve image contrast. One can easily see anatomy or pathology easily. Sometimes misregistration occurs in subtraction images, which can be rectified by pixel shift. Radiology needs quantitative imaging with measurements. This is possible by defining *region of interest* (ROI). The ROI may have multiple pixels. The mean value of all pixels may be assigned to that ROI. It has clinical application in bone mineral study, calcified lung nodule detection, and renal stone identification, including disease characteristics.

Edge enhancement is a software by which contrast of the edge can be increased. It has to satisfy two conditions, first the part should be fully exposed, secondly its SNR must be low. Otherwise noise can be enhanced along with edge enhancement. Smoothening is a software function by which image noise is reduced. Noise lies in the high frequency domain of the histogram. Adjusting the high frequency, noise can be eliminated. Equalization is the technique in which underexposed region is made darker and over exposed region is made lighter. Though this appears with lower contrast, it is useful to identify dense and lucent structures.

RECORDING OF DIGITAL IMAGE

Medical digital image can be printed directly using printers from the display monitors. The printers used in radiology may be divided into nonlaser and laser types. Nonlaser includes video monitor, thermal print heads, or inject technology. Laser printers are further divided into wet laser and dry laser category. Wet laser basically uses chemicals like darkroom film processing. In this, the film is exposed to a laser beam that modulates the image; later film is subjected to developing, fixing, and washing. This technology is now phasing out. Dry laser employs laser-induced thermal technology. A typical laser printer consists of the following parts:
- Electronic data
- Corona wires
- Photoreceptor drum
- Laser and mirror
- Ink roller
- Paper tray
- Fuser unit.

During the printing, the computer sends large number of electronic data of the order of few megabytes to the printer. The electronic circuit in the printer analyzes the above data and plans how it should appear correctly on the page. This electronic circuit in the printer resembles a small computer. The electronic circuit also activates a corona wire, which is a high voltage wire. It can give static electricity to anything nearby. A photoreceptor drum is kept nearby, which gains positive charge from the corona wire. Thus, the drum gains positive charge spread uniformly across its surface.

The electronic circuit also activates the laser which can draw the image of the paper onto the drum. The laser is not moving, instead the beam falls on a mirror and the mirror scans over the drum. The laser erases the positive charge in the drum and creates area of negative charge. Gradually, the image of the page is built up in the drum. The area of positive charge appears as white, whereas areas of negative charge appear as black. An ink roller touching the drum coats it with powdered

162　Medical X-ray Film Processing

ink (toner). The tonner is basically positively charged. When the toner and drum is in contact, the toner gives ink to the drum, only to the area where negative charge is present. No ink is attracted to the drum area where positive charge is present. Thus, an inked page of the drum is developed.

A sheet of paper from the hopper is feed forward to the drum. As the paper moves forward, uniform positive charge is given to the paper by another corona wire. Therefore, the positively charged paper attracts the negatively charged toner particles. Thus, the image of the drum is transferred into the paper, but the toner particles are resting lightly on the paper. The inked paper is passed on between two hot rollers, where the heat (120–140°C) and pressure permanently fix the toner particles into the paper. This makes the latent image into a permanent image. The final printout comes from the printer, still it is warm.

The following paragraph will explain step-by-step function of the laser printer (Fig. 8.7):

- Computer data of several MB reaches the printer (1).
- Printer electronic circuit plans how to print correctly the image (2).
- Printer electronic circuit activates the corona wire to give positive charge to the photoreceptor drum (3).
- The photoreceptor drum gets uniform positive charge across its surface (4).
- Printer electronic circuit makes laser and mirror to draw the page of the image on the drum. It makes area of negative charge on the drum (5).

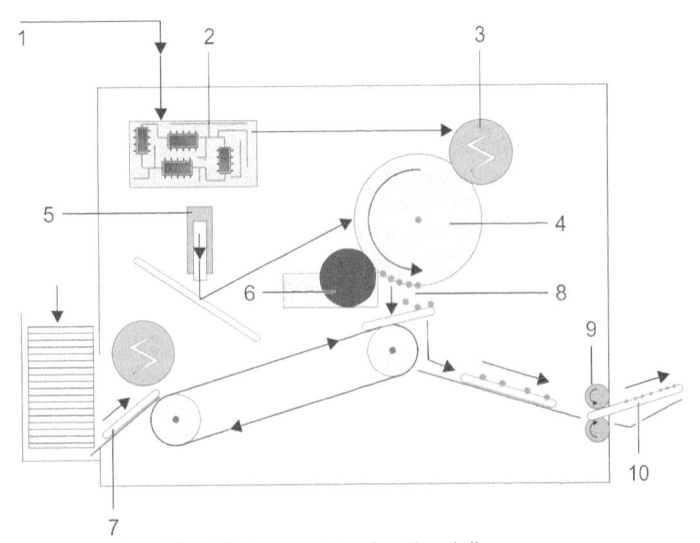

Fig. 8.7: Laser printer functional diagram.

Digital Radiography; Image Quality, Viewing, and Recording

- The ink roller touching the photoreceptor drum coats it with tiny particles of powdered ink, wherever area of negative charge is present (6).
- A positively charged paper is fed forward to the drum. The paper attracts tonner particles only from the area of the negative charge. Thus, image is transferred from the drum to the paper (7).
- The paper is moved between two hot rollers. The heat and pressure from the rollers fuse the toner particles in the paper permanently (8).
- The final printout comes out of the printer (9, 10).

The dry laser printers are basically made up of solid state technology and not involving any optical components. They are heat-sensitive, instead of light-sensitive. It uses multiple technologies, including radiographic, thermal, mechanical and digital process. It offers daylight loading facility. They provide printing for MRI, CT, DSA, picture archiving and communication system (PACS), computed radiography (CR) and DR systems. They offer high-resolution images with fast throughputs of multiformat multimodality printouts. A laser printer image may contain 325 pixels per inch. One can print 45–140 films per hour, depending on the film size. They are highly reliable, durable and user friendly. There is no wet process in this and no chemicals is involved. Hence, the size is small, occupies lesser space.

Advantages of hard copy:
- Films are instantly readable
- It can be prepared at any time
- Film is a physical record
- It makes physician job easier
- Films are not subjected to system failure
- Films cannot be corrupted like computer
- Serve the purpose of medicolegal cases.

Hard copy disadvantages:
- Involves high cost
- It is time consuming
- Printer is space occupying
- Films can be easily destroyed or lost
- Film may degrade image quality with storage.

Commercial Dry Laser Printers

The commercial dry laser printers that are used in hospital setup are shown in Figure 8.8A. They are basically DICOM-native imager, facilitates network connectivity easily. They provide 2–5 media sizes of different image sizes. The printing time is ultrashort, e.g. 75 sheets/hr for a size of 14 × 17 inch. Thus, it can handle 11 × 14 inch (86 sheets/hr) and 8 × 10 inch (140 sheets/hr), and enhance throughput. A 10 × 12 inch film imager may have 3070 × 3653 pixels of diagnostic area. The minimum printing resolution of 32 PPi (pixels per inch) and contrast resolution of 12 bits can be achieved.

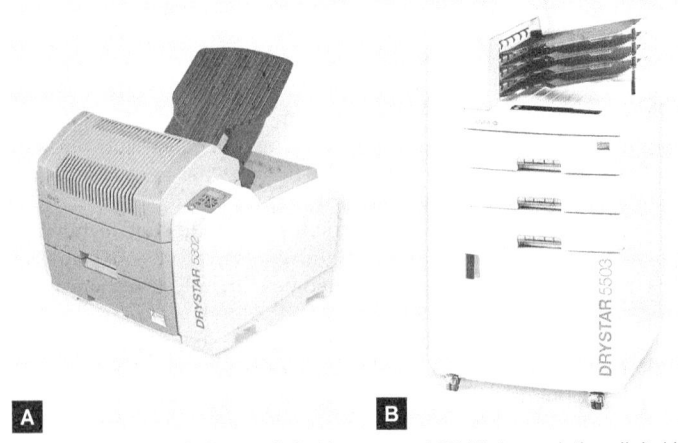

Figs. 8.8A and B: (A) Direct digital imager and (B) High-resolution digital imager. (*Courtesy*: Agfa Healthcare India Pvt. Ltd.)

Multiple media size direct digital imager (Fig. 8.8B) is also available. They have multiformat architecture, sorting function, and take printing work from different sources. Thus, the imager is capable of printing CT, MRI, DSA, digital radiography (CR and DR) and digital mammography images.

X-ray Film Viewer

X-ray films and digital image printout films are examined by using a viewing light box (Figs. 8.9A and B). While reading the X-ray film on the view box, magnification and external light influences the information. Use of low-ambient light and restricting light from the surroundings of the view box, will improve its performance. A typical view box consists of a light source of variable intensity. It is fitted in an aluminum box with glass or acrylic front screen.

Initially, ordinary light bulbs/tube lights of multiple numbers are used to match the view box size. Off late light-emitting diode (LED) lamp is used, which can serve to 200,000 hours, longer than the cold cathode fluorescent (CCFL) lamp. The light intensity can be varied from 300 cd/m^2 to 4500 cd/m^2, in order to reduce eye's fatigue. Generally, this is achieved by ON/OFF individual switch, with feather touch dimmer. The light source should spread the light uniformly on the screen, without any dark spot. It can provide nine digital grades to adjust brightness, to view different density of X-ray films.

It is fitted with automatic film sensor. When the film is inserted, it starts working and turns off automatically, while the film is removed. In

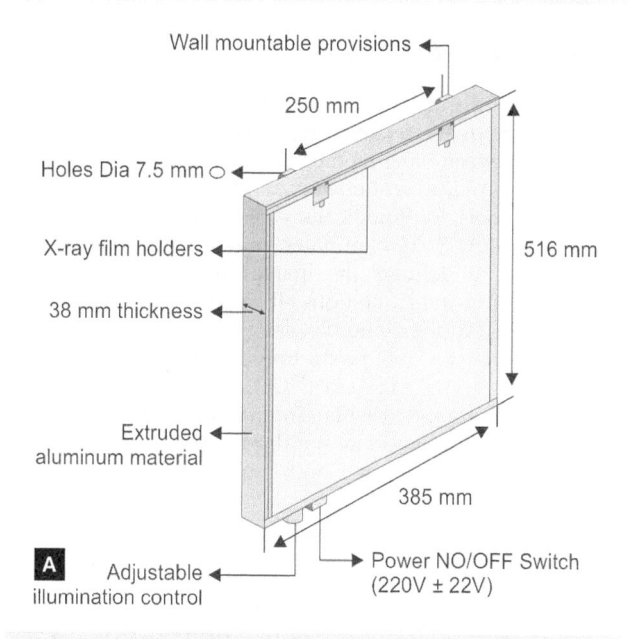

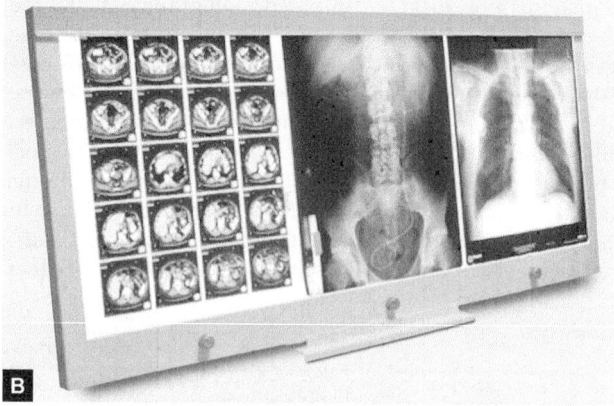

Digital Radiography; Image Quality, Viewing, and Recording 165

Figs. 8.9A and B: View box for X-ray films.

addition, it has close timer function, brightness memory function, etc. The close timer function will help to save power. When it works continuously for more than an hour, it will switch OFF automatically. The film viewer can remember the brightness; if the film is inserted again, it will show the same brightness. There is no need of brightness adjustment again. It is available in different sizes to read single or multiple or multiformat films. It has holders for X-ray films and wall mounting facility.

PICTURE ARCHIVING AND COMMUNICATION SYSTEM

The picture archiving and communication system (PACS) is a provision, used in medical imaging technology. It is an electronic network for communication between imaging modalities, display stations and image storage facility. It provides cost effective and easy access to images from multiple imaging tools. Radiological images and reports are transmitted digitally through PACS. It eliminates manual filing, retrieving and transport of films. It delivers the images timely and provides easy access to images and interpretations. It avoids traditional film based image retrieval, distribution and display. DICOM (*digital imaging and communications in medicine*, 1983) is the universal format for image storage and transfer, which is used in PACS. DICOM standard permits exchange of images among modalities, display monitors and storage devices. The present DICOM is an international standard. PACS is divided into image acquisition, display and storage and require following components namely:

- Imaging device (CR/DR/CT/MRI/US)
- Network system
- Work station
- Storage.

The imaging tools include computed radiography, digital radiography, CT, ultrasound, MRI and PET etc. The images from the modalities are sent to the Quality assurance (QA) work station, called PACS gateway (Fig. 8.10). A gate way is a computer system for connecting one network to other. It checks the patient demographics as well as attributes of the study. If the study information is correct, images are then passed to the archive for storage. Then the radiologists review the images through their workstations and make the final report. The workstation and archive is a bidirectional transmission. The patient's information, report and images are stored as an electronic file. These files can be viewed by other work

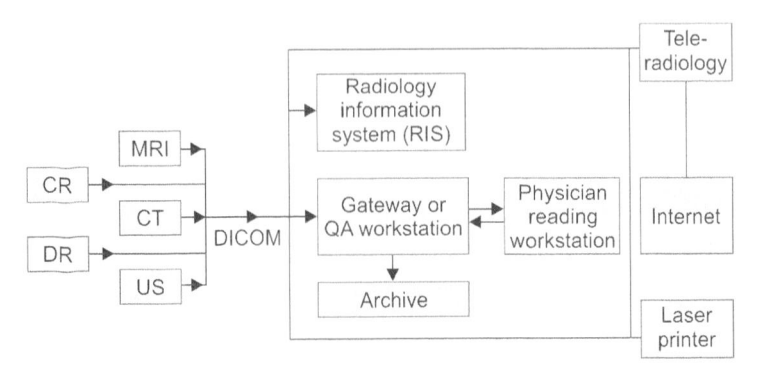

Fig. 8.10: Picture archiving and communication system, block diagram.

stations through *Tele radiology* services. Even a radiologist outside the hospital can access the image, under permission.

PACS uses web-based interfaces to use internet or *wide area network* (WAN) as their way of communication, via virtual private network (VPN) or secure sockets layer (SSL). The client side software includes Activex, Java script and Java Applet. Very good pack up for patient images is required, in case of loss of images from PACS. Hence, the images are automatically sending their copies to a separate computer for storage. PACS should be integrated with *Radiology information system* (RIS) and *Hospital information system* (HIS).

The PACS finds variety of uses as given below:
- It replaces hard copy such as films
- Provides rapid retrieval and remote access, including distance education and Tele-radiology,
- Provides electronic image integration platform with easy access to HIS (hospital information system), RIS (Radiology information system)
- Improves operation efficiency and manages radiology workflow, such as patient examinations
- Reduce time and financial cost, but involves initial capital cost
- Eliminates loss and misplacement of image, which is common in film.

Tele-Radiology

Tele-radiology (TR) is the transmission of patient images from one location to another location. The images include X-ray, CT, ultrasound and MRI etc. The main purpose is to share the images or study with other radiologists and physicians. Since the number of radiologists is lesser than the imaging procedures, Tele-radiology fills the shortage of radiologists.

Tele-radiology uses internet, telephone, *wide area network* (WAN) and *local area network* (LAN). Specialized software is used to transmit images. The internet uses high *transmission control protocol* (TCP) and *internet protocol* (IP). The TCP spilt the information into small packets, so that it can be moved through internet. *World Wide Web* (www) refers the collection of computers that exchange information by using an internet. It uses *hypertext transfer protocol* (HTTP). If the image data is larger, then it requires image compression. It can be done either with lossless or lossy compression. Advanced technologies such as graphic processing, voice recognition, and image compressions are used in Tele-radiology.

Tele-radiology improves patient care, by allowing radiologist services, who are physically not present at that location. This is highly true in specialist such as MR Radiologist or Neuro-radiologist, or Periodic radiologist, etc., who are available only in urban cities. Tele-radiology allows round the clock service of the specialists without interruption.

OPTIMAL IMAGE QUALITY IN DIGITAL RADIOGRAPHY

Computed Radiography

Computed radiography digital system uses exposure indicators namely, *sensitivity* (S), *exposure index* (EI) and *log mean* (lgM). The S is inversely proportional to the exposure of the imaging plate, e.g. 200 S = 1 mR radiation exposure. The optimal value of S varies from 250–300 for torso and 75–125 for extremity (**Fuji, Philips, Konica**). The EI is directly proportional the exposure of imaging plate (**Philips, Kodak**). The optimal value of EI ranges from 1800–1900 for buchy related procedures. Changes in EI of the order of 300 will double the detector exposure. Some vendors use lgM number, which is proportional to the detector exposure. Since the above number is logarithmic, change of number, say 0.3, will double the exposure. The optimal value in this system is 1.9–2. When a CR cassette is exposed within the accepted range of S or EI or lgM, then image is adjusted for contrast and brightness. If the cassette is exposed outside range of the exposure factors, may result in noisy image, not suitable for interpretation. The radiologic technician should select the suitable anatomical part and projection before each processing, so that the computer may use suitable histogram.

Digital Radiography

The digital radiography (DR) systems uses *dose-Area-Product* (DAP) meter, that is embedded in the collimator. The DAP value is expressed in cGy-m^2 and it depends on exposure factors and field size. It indicates the patient dose as well as the volume of tissue irradiated. Attempts have been made to unify the exposure values in digital systems. Hence, terms like *exposure index* (EI), *target exposure index* (EIT) and *deviation index* (DI) are recommended. The EI refers the exposure at the detector level, which is controlled by the SNR. The EI is directly proportional to mAs, when kV is kept constant. The EIT refers the exposure at the target (anatomy) level, which will vary anatomywise. DI is the deviation between the exposure index and target exposure index (EI -EIT). Thus, the DI will tell the deviation from the ideal value, for a given anatomical part.

Speed Class

In screen-film radiography system, speed is used, which refers the required exposure to obtain desired density. Since, digital systems have wide dynamic range, use of speed is inaccurate and should be avoided. Here, the term *speed class* is used, which indicates the exposure level for an optimal image. Speed class refers to exposure level at which the system is operated and it is related to DQE. A digital system can be operated to any speed class. It affects only the quantum mottle, not the brightness. As the speed class increases, the image noise also increases. As the speed class

Digital Radiography; Image Quality, Viewing, and Recording

decreases, patient dose increases. Hence, a balanced approach is required to get a good quality image.

Influence of mAs

In screen-film system radiography, mAs control the density, which is no more valid in digital radiography. In addition, both image capture and display is done by the film. In DR, these functions are separate, the detector captures the image and the computer controls the density. However, the patient dose is controlled by the mAs. Use of high mAs leads to higher patient dose, and low mAs leads to noise image. In screen-film radiography, higher mAs is always recommended to avoid retakes. This concept totally fails in digital radiography.

Influence of kVp and Look up Table

In screen-film system, kVp controls contrast. In DR system, the look up tables (UT) controls the image contrast. DR computer uses UT in the form of histogram of luminance values. These values are used to evaluate the input intensities and assign predetermined gray scale values, which is called *rescaling*. Rescaling refers the computer adjustment to present the image in a pre-determined brightness. Therefore, overexposed detector image can be made lighter or underexposed may be made darker, by using computer rescaling.

Since the look up table controls the contrast, use of high kV (>15%) is recommended. This may facilitate use of lower mAs, resulting in lower patient dose. However, use of high kV leads to more scatter radiations, resulting in loss of image contrast. Digital radiography is more sensitive to scatter radiations, and scatter control is very important, than in screen–film systems. Hence, effective collimation and use of grid will reduce scatter radiation.

Over all, the digital radiography systems are not controlled by kVp and mAs, in terms of contrast and density as in the case of screen-film systems. Hence, high kVp and lower mAs are always recommended in DR, provided the scatter is under control. Use of grid and collimation will bring down scatter radiation and improve image quality. Though post processing improves image density and brightness, it is not true always, in all images. A poorly acquired image cannot be processed to the level of acceptance and interpretation.

9
Digital Radiography; Image Artifacts and Quality Assurance

IMAGE ARTIFACTS

An artifact in an image is something that does not correlate with the physical properties of the human body structure. It may obscure normal or abnormal structure or confound further interpretations. Understanding the mechanism of formation of artifacts may help to resolve or prevent their presence in the image appearance. This will improve not only the consistency, but also the radiographic quality. The artifact may affect the quality of patient care. Hence, attempts must be made to identify type and nature of artifacts in digital radiography. It is necessary to have strict quality control and institutional guidelines on artifacts.

Artifact does occur in screen-film radiography, similar way it also present in digital radiography. In digital radiography, digital images are produced by computed radiography (CR) and digital radiography (DR). Both systems use phosphor in the form of imaging plate and flat panel, respectively. The image processing algorithm and settings are different in each system. Hence, the type and causes of artifacts are different in both CR and DR, since the nature of image capture is different in each system. Generally, artifacts are divided into two broad categories:
- Image acquisition artifacts
- Image processing artifacts.

Some artifacts are unique to each system. However, artifacts due to image processing may be common in both systems. Let us discuss the digital radiography artifacts first and computed radiography artifacts later.

DIGITAL RADIOGRAPHY ARTIFACTS

Digital radiography employs flat panel systems for image capture either indirectly or directly. The signal detection and processing is different from computed radiography. Some artifacts are easy to identify and some of them may be seen on retrospective viewing. Some artifacts are subtle in nature, not able to identify easily. They can be viewed only during quality control tests. The artifact arises from the digital radiography (flat panel systems) are summarized as follows:
- *Detector mishandling artifacts*:
    - Detector drops
    - Liquid contamination
- *Image acquisition technique artifacts*:
    - Back scatter
    - Image saturation

Digital Radiography; Image Artifacts and Quality Assurance

- *Flaws in detector calibration/limitations artifacts*:
  - Detector calibration limitation
  - Inverse focal spot and calibration
  - Flawed detector calibration
  - Evolving detector defect
  - Failure of detector offset correction
- *Image processing artifacts*:
  - Electronic shutter failure
  - Poor identification of values of interest
  - Midgray clipping
  - Metal interface artifacts
  - Grid-line suppression failure.

Detector Mishandling Artifacts

If the detector is dropped from the hand, it may disturb the readout electronics or change the gain and offset. It will appear as narrow white band, which may grow over a period of time. It may appear in the form of smooth edge defect and vertical lines (Fig. 9.1). It may also be seen as large area of signal dropout with rounded perimeter or white speckles. In such cases, the detector needs to be calibrated or removed from use.

Detector with liquid contamination may show banding in the image (Fig. 9.2). Detectors which are not sealed properly may absorb water from the patient's water mattress. This water may enter into the detector and damage the readout electronics. Hence, detector must be covered with plastic bag and sealed, to avoid liquid drop artifacts.

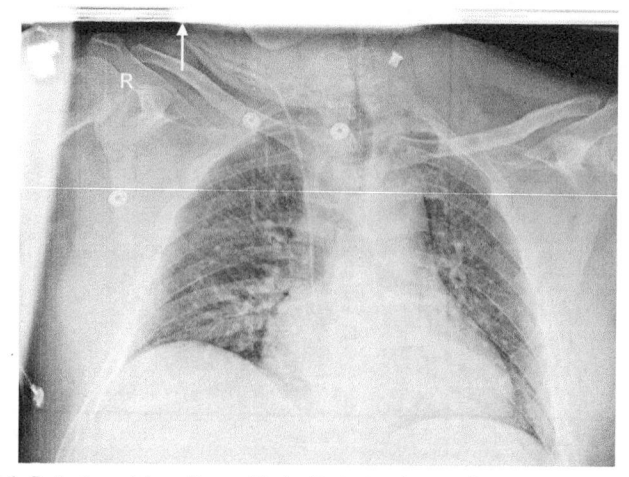

Fig. 9.1: Detector mishandling artifacts: Detector drop artifact appear as white band (arrow) at the top of the chest radiograph.
(*Courtesy*: Alisa I. Walz-Flannigan et al, Radiographics 2018)

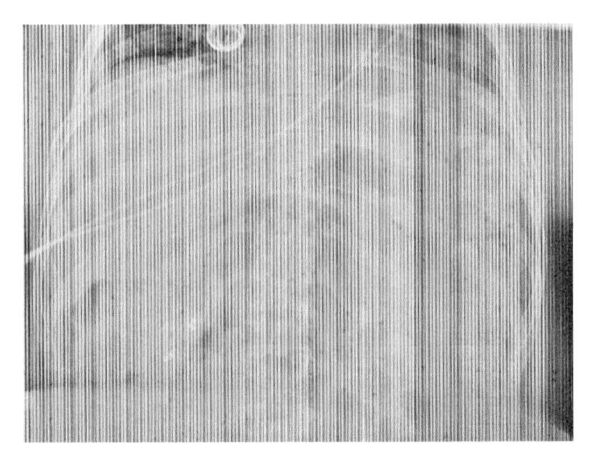

Fig. 9.2: Detector mishandling artifacts: Liquid contamination artifact appear as repeated vertical banding in a chest radiograph.
(*Courtesy*: Alisa I. Walz-Flannigan et al, Radiographics 2018)

Image Acquisition Technique Artifacts

Radiation incident at the backside of the detector get scattered back, leads to back scatter artifacts. The back scattered radiation reaches the detector elements and shows the shadow of the detector electronics (Fig. 9.3). The detector electronics may be superimposed on the image. This is common with big body size and wide collimator opening or in certain imaging

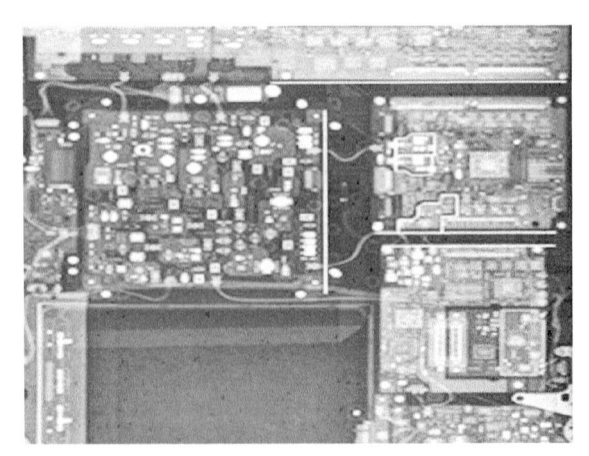

Fig. 9.3: Image acquisition technique artifacts: Back scatter artifact shows the shadow of detector electronics.
(*Courtesy*: Alisa I. Walz-Flannigan et al, Radiographics 2018)

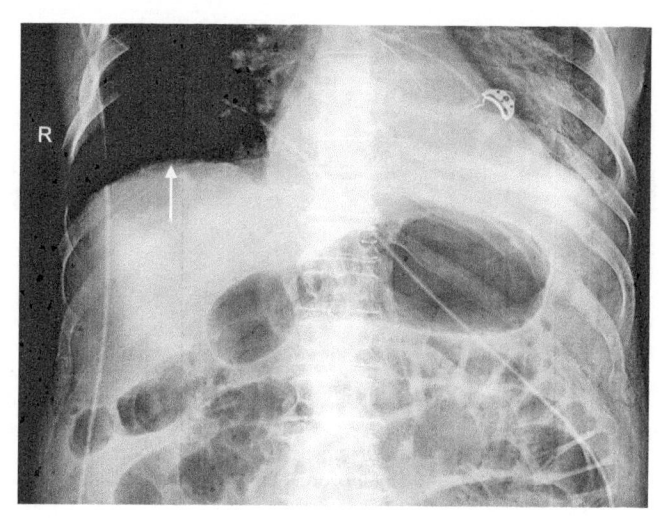

Fig. 9.4: Image acquisition technique artifacts: Image saturation artifact showing loss of image (arrow), due to excessive exposure.
(*Courtesy*: Alisa I. Walz-Flannigan et al, Radiographics 2018)

geometries, where the scatter is more. This can be avoided by proper tight collimation, good imaging geometry or providing lead at the back of the detector to remove back scatter.

If the exposure is greater than the dynamic range of the receptor or image processing algorithm, image saturation artifacts may appear. It may lead to over exposure and anatomy will be missed (Fig. 9.4). Usually, it appears in stimulated grid acquisition technique, where algorithm is used to suppress scatter, instead of physical grid. The saturation point of DR is much lower than CR. Hence, it is more likely in flat panel systems, compared to CR. To avoid this the patient's size and source to detector distance should be measured. Size specific techniques should be employed.

Flaws in Detector Calibration/Limitation Artifacts

The detector calibration limitation artifacts appear as vertical stripping in the area of raw radiation. The lines appear in the background on the image, without involving the anatomy (Fig. 9.5). This may arise when the exposure exceeds the gain and offset corrections of the detector calibration. Use of optimized target exposure technique and education of technologists may avoid such artifacts.

Presence of debris in the X-ray beam creates inverse focal spot and calibration artifacts. This may appear as trapezoidal opacity surrounded by magnified areas of lucency (Fig. 9.6). This is due to either removal of

174 Medical X-ray Film Processing

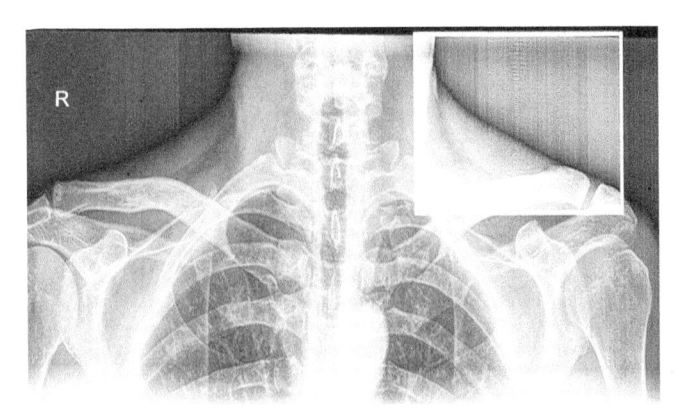

Fig. 9.5: Flaws in detector calibration artifacts: Shows vertical lines in the background at the raw radiation part of the image.
(*Courtesy*: Alisa I. Walz-Flannigan et al, Radiographics 2018)

Fig. 9.6: Flaws in detector calibration artifacts: Inverse focal spots and calibration artifact shows trapezoidal opacity, which is the pinhole image of the focal spot caused by lead debris near the X-ray tube.
(*Courtesy*: Alisa I. Walz-Flannigan et al, Radiographics 2018)

collimator or presence of lead debris near the X-ray tube. This can be avoided by removing the debris, calibrating the detector and collimator adjustment.

Flawed detector calibration artifacts appear as irregular lines, which is radiolucent. It is in a fixed position, irrespective of detector rotation. Presence of any external device in the field of view during the detector

Digital Radiography; Image Artifacts and Quality Assurance

Fig. 9.7: Evolving detector effect artifact: Shows several trapezoidal inverse focal spot artifacts along with many bloblike artifacts.
(*Courtesy*: Alisa I. Walz-Flannigan et al, Radiographics 2018)

calibration may create this type of artifacts, e.g. pillow edge. To avoid this, recalibration of detector or validation of detector calibration with flat field image can be performed.

Evolving detector defect is a subtle artifact seen only during quality control testing. It appears as blob like areas of opacity (Fig. 9.7). It remains stationary during detector rotation. It will not change in size with source to image distance. It is due to formation of bubbles between the layers of the scintillator and thin film transistor (TFT) of the detector. Recalibration of the detector may avoid such artifacts.

Failure of detector calibration offset artifacts appear as superimposed inverse image from previous acquisition. This may be caused by the failure of detector offset calibration after the change of battery. Avoiding the battery change during the procedure may help to avoid such artifacts.

Image Processing Artifacts

Electronic shutter failure artifact arises from incorrect collimation. As a result the collimator may fail to detect the anatomy (Fig. 9.8), leading to poor electric shuttering. The procedure may be repeated, re-shuttering and reprocessing, to avoid such artifacts.

Poor identification of values of interest artifact shows the appearance of washed out images (Fig. 9.9). It gives the impression of under exposure, even though higher exposure is given. The image can be reprocessed with smaller areas of interest to avoid such artifacts.

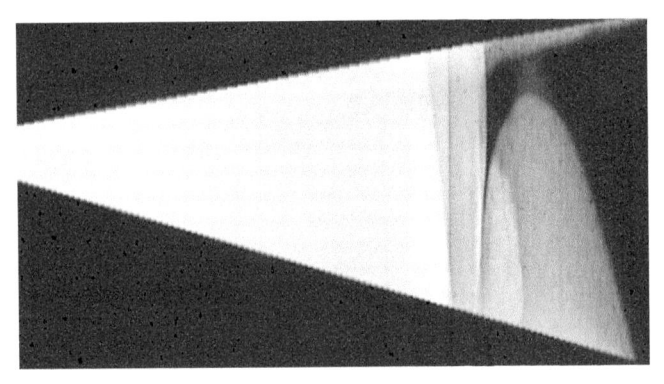

Fig. 9.8: Image processing artifacts: Electronic shutter failure artifact-lateral hip radiograph shows failed detection of collimator edges and poor electronic shuttering. (*Courtesy*: Alisa I. Walz-Flannigan et al, Radiographics 2018)

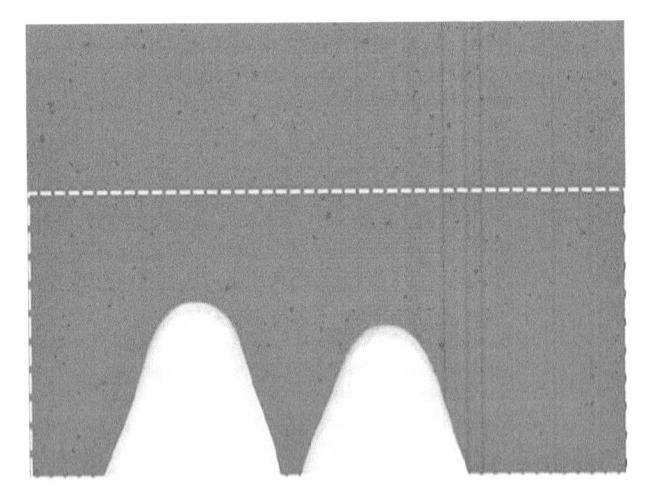

Fig. 9.9: Image processing artifacts: Poor identification of values of interest artifact-A patella radiograph seen as washed out, similar to underexposure. (*Courtesy*: Alisa I. Walz-Flannigan et al, Radiographics 2018)

Midgray clipping artifacts arise in the form of loss of detail in the cement and cement-implant boundary (Fig. 9.10). It is due to poor optimization of signal equalization processing (contrast enhancement). Adjustment of processing setting or option of processing with small field of view may avoid such artifacts.

Metal interface artifact appears in bone-metal interface, suggesting a false lucency. It is related to excessive edge enhancement, suggestive

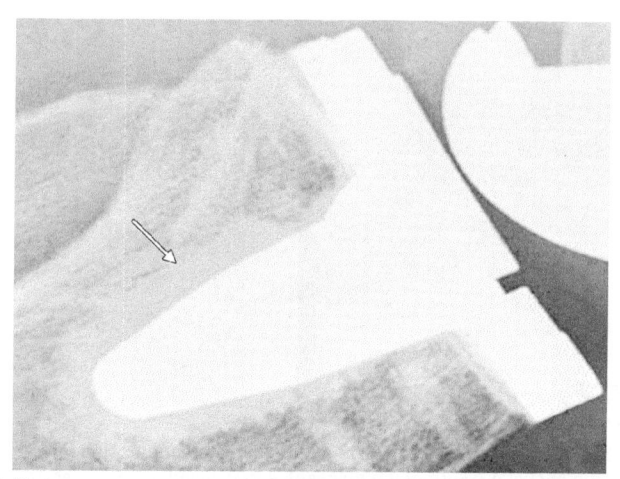

Digital Radiography; Image Artifacts and Quality Assurance

Fig. 9.10: Image processing artifacts: Midgray clipping artifact-knee radiograph showing homogeneous gray appearance of the cement with loss of detail.
(*Courtesy*: Alisa I. Walz-Flannigan et al, Radiographics 2018)

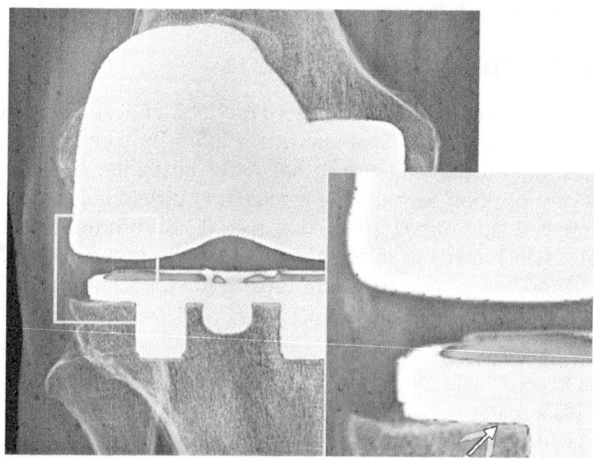

Fig. 9.11: Image processing artifacts due to metal interface: Knee radiograph shows false lucency as well as stair stepped edge that does not related to the structure of the imaged object, at the metal-bone interface.
(*Courtesy*: Alisa I. Walz-Flannigan et al, Radiographics 2018)

of loosening in the implant (Fig. 9.11). Alternate processing setting may eliminate lucency artifacts.

Grid-line suppression failure artifact shows grid-line on the radiograph, which is due to failure of grid-line suppression algorithm

178 Medical X-ray Film Processing

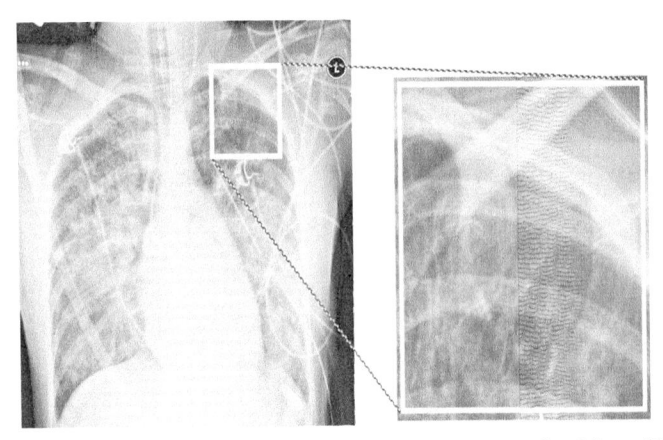

Fig. 9.12: Image processing artifacts due to grid-line suppression failure: Chest radiograph shows a failure of the grid lines suppression software (square box). (*Courtesy*: Alisa I. Walz-Flannigan et al, Radiographics 2018)

(Fig. 9.12). Proper function of grid-line suppression algorithm must be ensured to avoid such artifacts.

COMPUTED RADIOGRAPHY ARTIFACTS

Computed radiography was introduced in 1983 and still widely used in various hospitals. It is a cost-effective solution to convert screen-film radiography into a digital setup. It has lot of flexibility; cassette can be placed at any position, cassette are available in different sizes and more suitable for bed side radiography. However, it also produces artifacts in the images, which leads to misdiagnosis, especially in medicolegal cases. Computed radiography artifacts are broadly divided into the following category:

- *Acquisition artifacts*:
    - Object
    - Back scatter
    - Grid use
    - Over/under exposure
- *Software or image processing artifacts*:
    - Dirt or dust
    - Imaging plate damage
    - Dead lines
- *Signal processing artifacts*:
    - Bad plate erasure
    - Saturation
    - Shading correction

- *Signal transmission artifacts*:
  - Readout failure
- Image processing artifacts.

Explaining the above said artifacts, their causes and remedy is beyond the scope of this book. However, attempts are being made to show some of the artifacts that everybody is facing in the clinics (Figs. 9.13 to 9.17).

Image receptor should be kept clean. Any dust in the image plate (IP) or in the CR mirror and lens system can cause artifacts. Scratches or

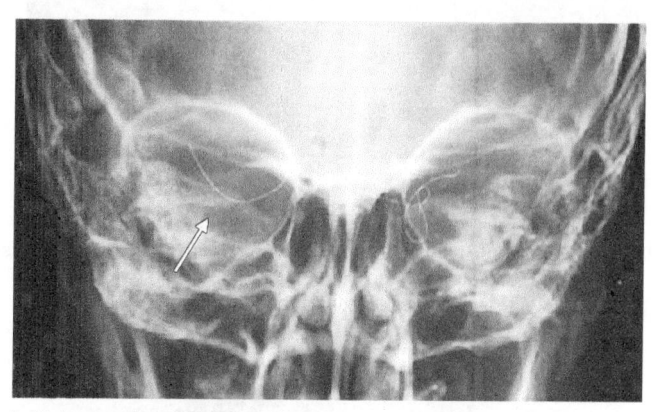

Fig. 9.13: Image plate (IP) artifacts, caused by a hair cling to IP during the skull image.
(*Courtesy*: LJ Cesar et al. BJR 2001)

Fig. 9.14: Image plate (IP) artifacts: A crack (arrow) in IP looks like a foreign body.
(*Courtesy*: LJ Cesar et al. BJR 2001)

180 Medical X-ray Film Processing

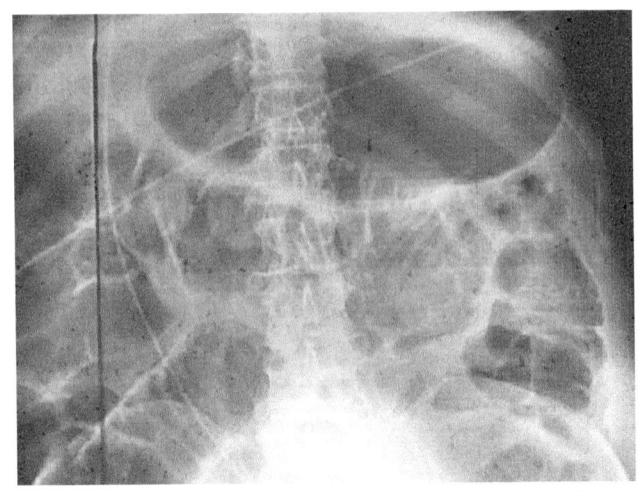

Fig. 9.15: Image plate (IP) artifacts: The dark vertical line is caused by backscattered radiation transmitted through the back of the cassette.
(*Courtesy*: LJ Cesar et al. BJR 2001)

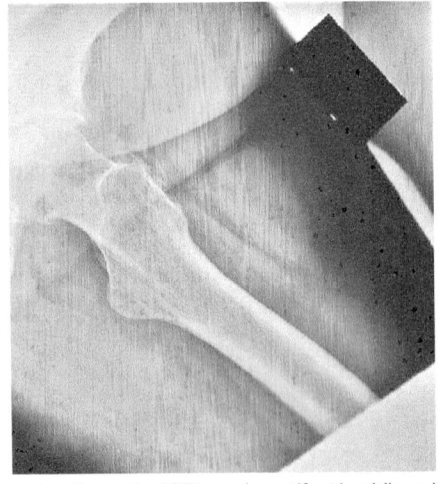

Fig. 9.16: Computed radiography (CR) reader artifact in oblique hip view: Malfunction of the electronic board that controls the photomultiplier tube in the reader. (*Courtesy*: LJ Cesar et al. BJR 2001)

malfunction of pixels can also cause artifacts. Imaging plate is susceptible for cracking, which may start from the middle of the plate. Debris present in the IP may prevent emission of light during laser scanning. The resultant image may appear bright. Since IP has high sensitivity to scatter radiation,

Digital Radiography; Image Artifacts and Quality Assurance

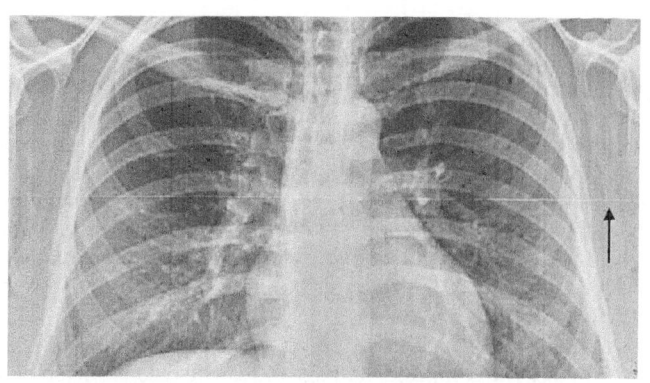

Fig. 9.17: Computed radiography (CR) reader artifact: A horizontal white line (arrow) caused by dirt on the light guide of the reader.
(*Courtesy*: LJ Cesar et al. BJR 2001)

backscattered radiation can cause artifacts. Generally, IPs are erased automatically after each radiograph. Incomplete erasure of the previous image appears as ghost image. A receptor not used too long, should be erased either manually or in the CR reader, before taking a new radiograph. For incorrect exposure, IPs are erased with long exposure cycle.

To overcome image receptor artifacts, the IP system should be cleaned regularly. Vendor's cleaning recommendations should be followed. The frequency of cleaning depends on the usage and workload. For cleaning, lint-free nonwoven cotton gauze (100% cotton) with lens cleaner is used. To start with, the IP surface is wiped off with dry gauze. If the stains are still present, the gauze is dampened with ethanol anhydride and the IP is cleaned, followed by dry cleaning. Such cleaning must be done in a zigzag way. Frequent cleaning with *ethanol anhydride* may cause yellowing of the IP edges.

The IPs must be stored under 35°, away from sunlight, ultraviolet, and radioactive sources. It should not be bent or subjected to any heavy force, e.g. dropping the IP on the floor or table. The damaged IPs should be isolated and not to be used for patient work. Another important precaution is that the IP is never scratched with technologist's nails and should not be moistened in water or chemicals.

Software artifact occurs during preprocessing and image compression. In preprocessing, dead pixel or row is a matter of concern. Then one has to use interpolation technique to assign a value for the dead pixels or rows. Correcting algorithm is available to do interpolation. Sometime, IP cassette is irradiated with X-ray beam, which can produce irregular pattern. To avoid this, *flat fielding* technique is performed. It is basically a software correction that makes all the pixels of uniform response.

IMAGE COMPRESSION

Digital radiography image occupies higher memory, therefore image field size is very high. In the case of 24 cm × 30 cm IP cassette used in mammography can occupy 50 MB field size per image. If multiple views are involved, the field size goes to few hundred MBs. There are difficulties in transmitting such images electronically for teleradiology or picture archiving and communication system (PACS). Hence, there is a need for image compression such as *lossless* and *lossy*. If the image is not compressed, failure may occur in electronic processing and the image cannot be interpreted.

Lossless compression can reduce the data file up to 10–50% of the original file size. The compressed image file can be reconstructed as same as the original file. This is most suitable for smaller image file, but not for larger image file. Lossy compression can reduce the file size to less than 10%. It is suitable for large field size, in which fine detail is not required. This is most suitable for teleradiology, but not for computer-aided diagnosis (CAD). Generally, CAD system uses uncompressed file to avoid compression artifacts.

Therefore, proper image processing is very important to avoid artifacts. At the same time image processing cannot correct everything (Figs. 9.18A and B).

Other artifact includes collimation, histogram selection, backscatter, and patient positioning. If the X-ray beam is not properly collimated, exposure field recognition errors may occur. The corresponding

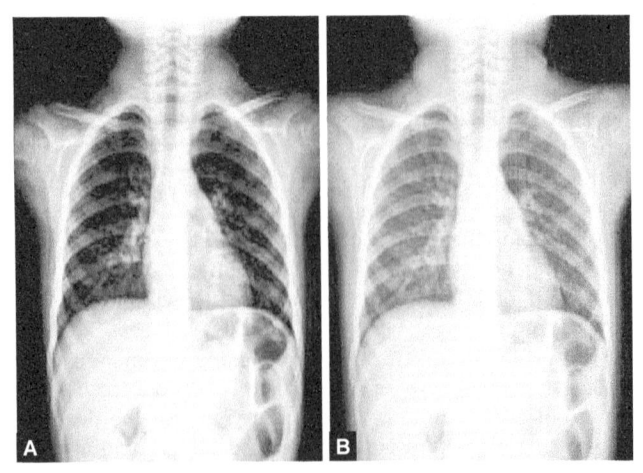

Figs. 9.18A and B: Image processing artifact: (A) Adult parameters are used for pediatric radiography due to vendor recommendations and (B) Modified image processing suggested by the user.

Digital Radiography; Image Artifacts and Quality Assurance

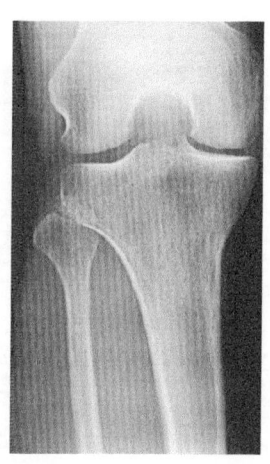

Fig. 9.19: Operator error artifact: Grid lines seen as moire pattern in the knee image, due to use of grid with low frequency lines. The grid lines are parallel to the laser scan lines. This can be avoided by using grid lines >60 lines/cm, so that the grid lines should be perpendicular to the scan lines.
(*Courtesy*: LJ Cesar et al. BJR 2001)

histogram may involve signal outside the X-ray field, resulting in artifacts. This may appear as very dark or light or noisy images. All these mostly arise from operator's error (Fig. 9.19). Therefore, technologists can create artifacts; they should be trained properly before handling digital systems. They should be aware of various artifacts and its causes and remedial measures.

In screen-film radiography, proper collimation reduces patient radiation dose and improves image contrast. Digital radiography provides the same, in addition to image histogram. Improper collimation may lead the histogram, improperly analyzed, and resulting in artifacts. Histogram-related artifacts can be avoided by proper collimation and centering. Generally, 2 or 4 X-ray exposure field is advised per imaging plate. Even in such cases, the collimated field should consist of proper separation and four distinct margins for each image. This can be achieved by shielding the unexposed area of each exposure, called *partitioning*. Exposure of 3 X-ray fields may be out of center and reduces image contrast, which can be avoided (Figs. 9.20 and 9.21). Few more interesting artifacts are shown in Figures 9.22A and B to 9.25A and B, which are self explanatory.

QUALITY CONTROL

Screen-film systems have been provided with quality control protocols to ensure quality of medical images. Similarly, digital imaging also requires

184 Medical X-ray Film Processing

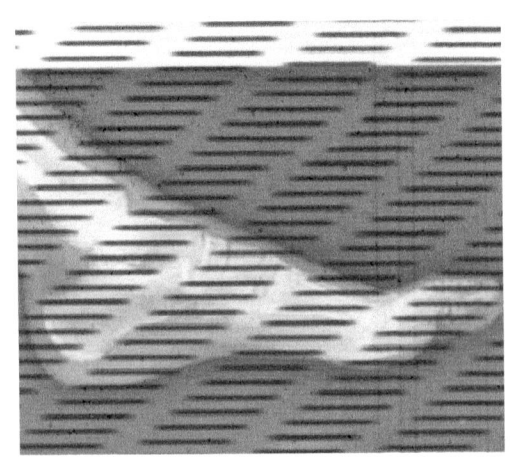

Fig. 9.20: Other artifacts: Missing lines or pixels in the computed radiography system, indicating memory problem.

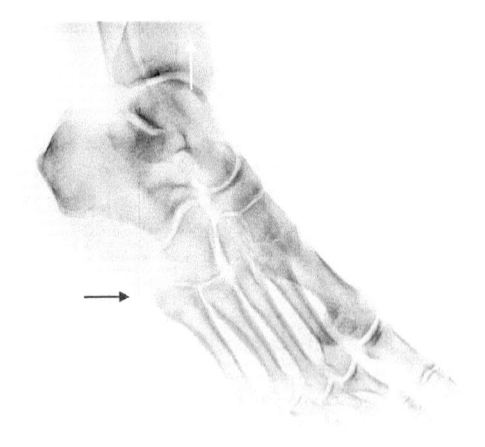

Fig. 9.21: Laser printer artifact in oblique foot: Vertical black line (black arrow) is due to laser printer and the horizontal black line (white arrow) is due to dirt on the light guide of the photo multiplier.
(*Courtesy*: LJ Cesar et al. BJR 2001)

quality control protocols. Lot of efforts has been undertaken by various agencies as listed below:
- The Society of Motion Pictures and Television Engineers (SMPTE)-RP133-1991
- National Electrical Manufacturers Association (NEMA)-DICON standard (PS3)

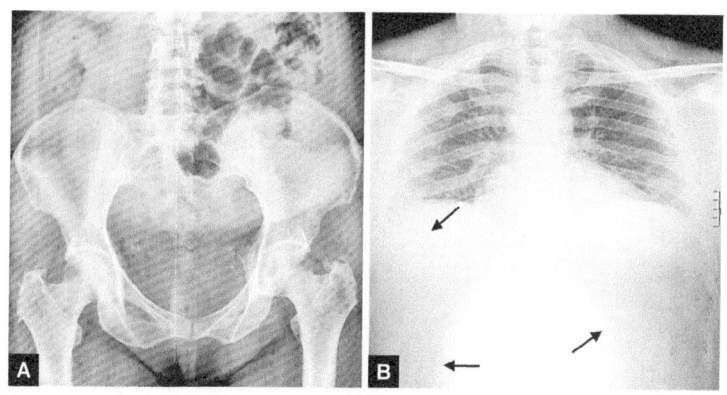

Figs. 9.22A and B: Computed radiography artifacts: (A) Improper grid usage with low grid frequency, image appears with moire pattern and (B) Light bulb effect, due to high kilo voltage used for obese patients or improper collimation.
(*Courtesy*: Chandrakant Manmath Shetty et al. AJR 2011)

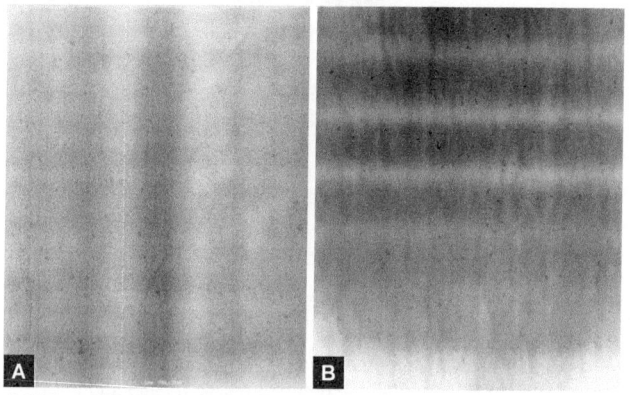

Figs. 9.23A and B: Computed radiography artifacts: (A) Reader roller damage and (B) Imaging plate Phosphor wear.
(*Courtesy*: Alisa Walz-Flannigan, Mayo Clinic, AAPM MEET, 2013)

- Deutsches Institut Fur Normung E.V (DIN) V 6868-57
- International Standards Organization (ISO) 9241 and 13406 series
- Video Electronics Standards Association (VESA)—flat panel display measurement standard
- American Association of Physicists in Medicine (AAPM) TG 18.

The AAPM Task Group (TG) 18 has developed set of test patterns and procedures (Figs. 9.26A to I), as given below:
- Geometric distortion
- Display reflection

186 Medical X-ray Film Processing

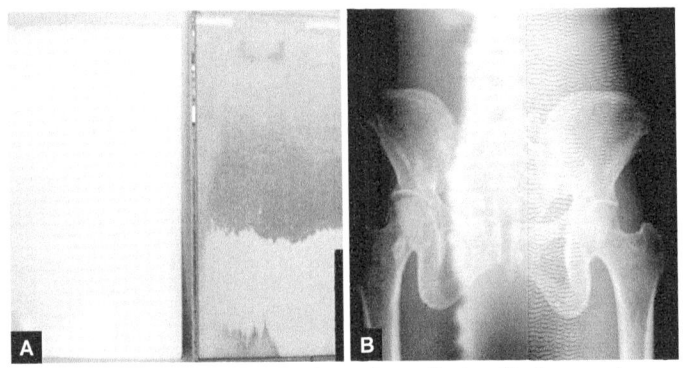

Figs. 9.24A and B: Computed radiography artifacts: (A) Damaged cassette-yellowing due to cleaning agent and (B) Phantom image shows the effect of damaged cassette, cassette needs to be withdrawn from further use.
(*Courtesy*: Alisa Walz-Flannigan, Mayo Clinic, AAPM MEET, 2013)

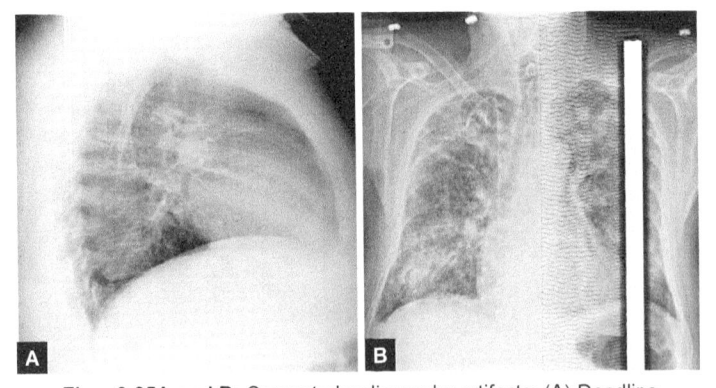

Figs. 9.25A and B: Computed radiography artifacts: (A) Deadline and (B) Readout failure, detector needs recalibration.
(*Courtesy*: Alisa Walz-Flannigan, Mayo Clinic, AAPM MEET, 2013)

- Luminance
- Luminance spatial and angular dependence
- Display resolution
- Display noise
- Veiling glare
- Display chromaticity.

Geometric Distortion

Geometric distortion arises from aberrations that cause the image, not similar to that of the original image. They are three kinds of distortions, namely:

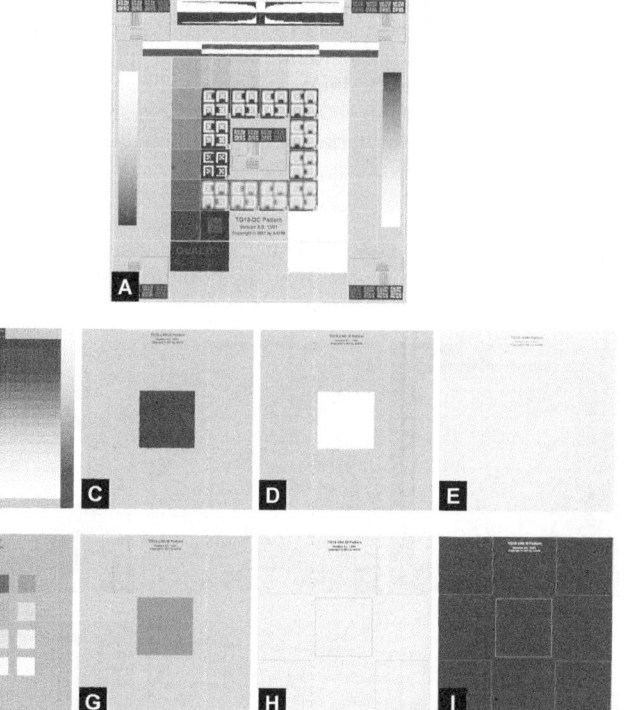

Figs. 9.26A to I: Quality assurance test pattern for evaluation of display characteristics: (A) TG18-QC; (B) TG18-PQC; (C) TG18-CT; (D) TG18-LN8-01; (E) TG18-LN8-08; (F) TG18-LN18-18; (G) TG18-UNL80; (H) TG18-UN80 and (I) TG18-UNL10 (AAPM TG18, 2005).

- Pincushion (concave distortion)
- Barrel (convex distortion)
- Skew distortion.

They are basically nonlinearity distortions within the active display area, which can cause local variations of image geometry. This can be directly related to the quality of the deflection coils and its electronics.

The first two distortions can be observed at the horizontal and vertical edges of the active area. Geometric distortions arise from improper setup of the display controller or mismatch between the display device and controller. Magnetic field can also cause geometric distortions in cathode-ray tube (CRT) devices. This can be compensated by the magnetic and electronic adjustments.

Geometric distortions can be assessed by both visual and quantitative evaluation by using the *AAPM TG18 QC* test patterns (Figs. 9.26J to R).

188 Medical X-ray Film Processing

The test pattern consists of multiple inserts embedded in a mid-pixel value background. This consists of number of gridlines and luminance patches. The test pattern should fill the entire display area and is viewed at a distance of 30 cm. The linearity pattern should be checked visually across the display area and at the edges. The lines should appear straight, without any curvature or variations. In addition, the lines should appear equally spaced.

Display Reflection

The luminance is the light generated by the display device. An ideal device should only have its own light luminance. In practice, room

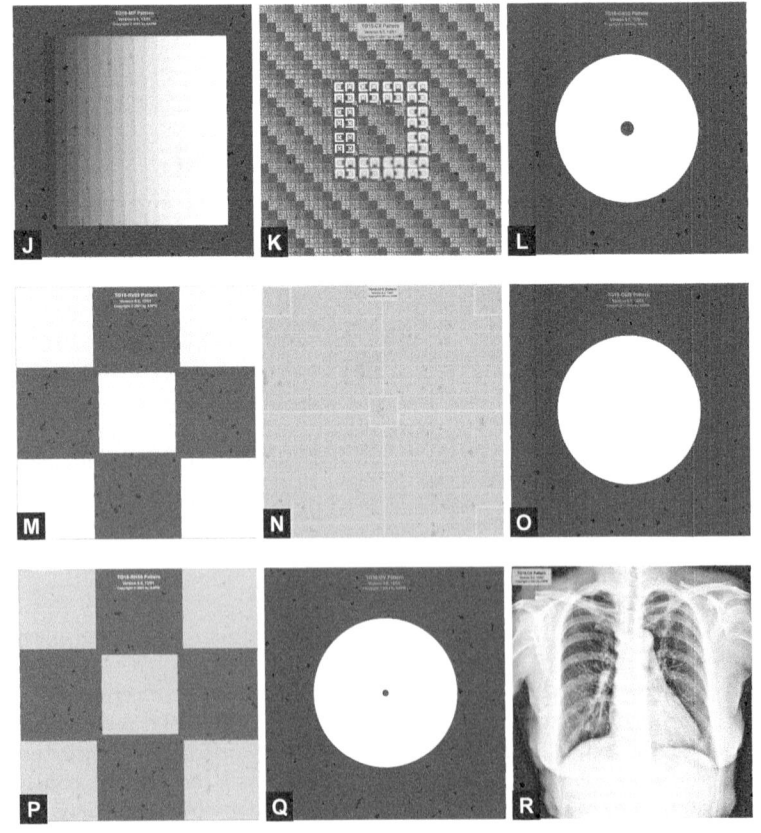

Figs. 9.26J to R: Quality assurance test pattern for evaluation of display characteristics: (J) TG18-MP, (K) TG18-RV89, (L) TG18-RH50, (M) TG18-CX, (N) TG18-AFC, (O) TG18-GV, (P) TG18-GA30, (Q) TG18-GQB, and (R) TG18-CH (AAPM TG18, 2005).

Digital Radiography; Image Artifacts and Quality Assurance

light gets reflected at the display source and add additional luminance to the device. Hence, the performance of the display device depends on its reflection characteristics. Therefore, there is need to evaluate the reflection characteristics of the system, in order to provide optimal room lighting (ambient illumination). The reflection has two forms, namely:
- Specular reflection
- Diffuse reflection.

Specular reflection is said to have occurred when the angle of incidence is equal to the angle of reflection. It provides virtual image of the light source, like a mirror. In diffuse reflection, the light is randomly scattered out and no virtual image of the source is produced. One can measure the specular reflection by using a small diameter source of diffuse white light, e.g. halogen spot lamp, with a glass diffuser at the exit surface. The light source should be brighter than 200 cd/m^2. The light source should be kept at 15° from the center of the display (Figs. 9.26S to U). The reflection spot luminance is measured. The specular reflection coefficient is the ratio of the reflection spot luminance to that of directly viewed spot luminance. All the measurements should be carried out in a darkroom.

Luminance Response

The luminance response of a display device is the relation between displayed luminance and the input values of a standardized display system. The displayed luminance consists of both light produced by the display system and the reflected ambient light. The light produced by the device has variable luminance from minimum to maximum. To measure luminance *TG18-CT* low-contrast pattern can be used. The pattern consists of 16 adjacent regions of varying luminance from 8 to 248, embedded in a uniform background (Fig. 9.27). Each patch contains four small 10 × 10 corner patches, which have ± 4 pixel value differences from the background. At the center of each patch, there is a half-moon shape with two targets at ± 2 pixel value differences from the background.

The test pattern should be evaluated for the central half-moon targets and four low-contrast objects at the corners of each of 16 different

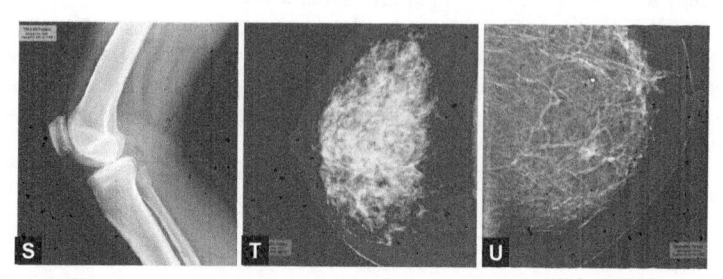

Figs. 9.26S to U: Quality assurance test pattern for evaluation of display characteristics: (S) TG18-KN, (T) TG18-MM1, and (U) TG18-MM2 (AAPM TG18, 2005).

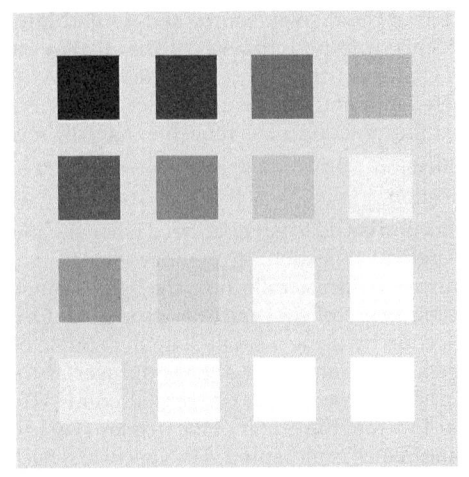

Fig. 9.27: AAPM TG18-CT test tool for the evaluation of contrast resolution, diffuse reflection, geometric distortion, luminance response and noise (AAPM TG18, 2005).

luminance regions. In addition, the bit-depth resolution of the display should be evaluated by using the *TG18-MP* test pattern. It should clearly demonstrate the low-contrast target at each of the 16 regions. This should be evaluated for horizontal contouring bands, their relative locations and grayscale reversals. All the above should be done at a viewing distance of 30 cm.

Luminance Spatial and Angular Dependence

The various discussions on luminance are based on perpendicular viewer. In practice it is not so; mostly it is viewed nonperpendicular angles. In that case, the display device exhibits spatial luminance nonuniformities and contrast variation, as a function of viewing angle. Luminance nonuniformity refers the maximum variation in luminance across the display area when a uniform pattern is displayed.

In the case of CRT monitors, the luminance decreases from the center to the edges and corners of the display. This is due to electron beam path length and landing angle and the face plate glass transmission characteristics. In the case of light-emitting diode (LED) systems, the causes are:
○ Backlight nonuniformity
○ Mura
○ Latent image
○ Spatial constancy of color coordinates
○ Thickness of the liquid crystal elements.

However, nonuniformities are lesser in LED display system.

Digital Radiography; Image Artifacts and Quality Assurance

Luminance nonuniformity can be measured while displaying a uniform pattern. It is quantified as the maximum relative luminance measurements. Spatial nonuniformity index can be obtained within 1 cm × 1 cm regions across the face plate divided by the mean value. The required test tools are *TG18-UN10* and *UN80*. The display devices suffer from variation in luminance as a function of viewing angle. The contrast ratio reduces with viewing angle both in horizontal and vertical orientations.

The variation of luminance of a display system can be quantified in terms of polar and azimuthal viewing angles. This can be used to determine the variation in luminance ratio as a function of viewing angle. The deviation of luminance response from the desired on-axis response can also be obtained as a function of viewing orientations. The viewing angle limitation should be labeled on the display device. The tool used for the test is *TG18-CT* pattern.

Display Resolution

Spatial resolution characteristics are very important, so that one can ensure that all the details are there in the displayed image. Insufficient resolution can compromise the accuracy of image interpretation. Resolution is often studied with modular transfer function (MTF), which is applicable to linear or quasi-linear imaging systems. If the display system has nonlinear luminance response, then it is critical. Hence, the display system response should be made linear first, then, the MTF is measured. To study this *TG18-QC or TG18-CX* test pattern can be used. The pattern must be displayed as one display pixel per image pixel. The resolution can be assessed visually by seeing the appearance of CX pattern. To quantify the MTF, one requires digital camera. It can capture a portion of the display and analyze the images.

Display Noise

Small and low-contrast objects are influenced by its size, contrast, and noise. The noise arises from superimposed noise and from intermediate surrounding noise. It is the high-frequency fluctuations/pattern, which interferes with the signal (< 1 cm). The display systems [CRT, active matrix liquid crystal display (AMLCD)] have inherent noise in the form of temporal and spatial components. This may be due to electronic conversion of video signal to photons and structured noise. Noise can also be caused by variations in uniformity of luminance.

Display systems spatial noise is described by the *normalized power spectrum* (NPS). It is normalized by the respective signal power. It is presented as 2D graph (spatial frequency vs NPS) along a particular direction. It is expressed in square millimeter by multiplying the normalized NPS by the area of the individual samples. Temporal noise can be studied with photomultiplier tube.

Veiling Glare

Light scattering in the display device induces a difference in luminance that veils the image. It is different from light reflection. In CRT system veiling glare arises from internal reflection of the electrons from Al layer, generation of secondary electrons in the phosphor and Al layer and the light scattering in the glass face plate. Veiling glare is measured by using a test pattern with a darkness surrounded by a bright field. There are only limited test patterns in the literature.

Display Chromaticity

Color tint may influence grayscale displays, used in the image workstation. It is affected by the balance of three primary colors forming the grayscale image. Color tint is affected by phosphor (CRT), spectrum of back light (AMLCD), and viewing angle (LCD). It is also an important factor in PACS acceptability. Visual color uniformity is performed by *TG18-UN80* test pattern. Quantitative assessment is done by *TG18-UNL80* test pattern.

Overall, the QC in digital radiography is very much important and it should be carried with suitable test tools. It is good to have a schedule for maintenance of IP plates and QC. The IP plates should be cleaned and inspected daily or quarterly basis. Plates should be erased every 48 hours, if unused. Every department should have identical processing codes, to enhance image quality. The required QC test should be carried out periodically (Table 9.1).

Table 9.1: Quality control test of various parameters of digital radiography, its frequency and test tools.

S.NO.	Parameter	Frequency	Test tool
1	General image quality and artifacts	Daily	TG-18-QC
2	Geometric distortion	Monthly or Quarterly	TG18-QC
3	Reflection	Monthly or Quarterly	TG18-AD
4	Luminance response	Monthly or Quarterly	TG18-LN01,TG18-LN08,TG18-LN18, & TG18-CT
5	Luminance dependence	Monthly or Quarterly	TG18-UNL10 & TG18-UNL80
6	Resolution	Monthly or Quarterly	TG18-QC &TG18-CX

10
Radiological Health and Safety

BIOLOGICAL EFFECTS OF RADIATION

Basically, the X-and gamma rays that are used in medicine are ionizing radiation of low linear energy transfer (LET) and low dose rate. The radiation enters the human body, interacts with water molecule, and produces radicals (OH*, H*). The radicals, in turn, interact with the *deoxyribonucleic acid* (DNA) molecule and produce mutation leading to cell death, cancer induction, and genetic and somatic effects. Sometimes the cell recovers its damage by its own ability and environment.

Ionizing radiation produces deterministic and stochastic effects (Figs. 10.1A and B). It can be early as well as late effects, either local or common in nature. A deterministic effect is one, which increases in severity with increasing absorbed dose in the affected individual, e.g. skin erythema, epilation, organ atrophy, fibrosis, cataract, blood changes, reduction of sperm count, etc. Deterministic effects are cell killings due to degenerative changes in the exposed individual. It has a threshold dose below which the effect is not seen. Its dose response curve is sigmoid in nature, likely to appear at higher dose (> 0.5 Gy). It is unlikely in medical exposure (diagnostic radiology and nuclear medicine), since it is a low-level exposure. Therefore, it is completely preventable.

Stochastic effect is one in which the probability of occurrence increases with increasing absorbed dose, rather than severity, e.g. carcinogenesis and genetic effect. The dose response for stochastic effect has no threshold and it is linear in nature. It is seen only at a later period

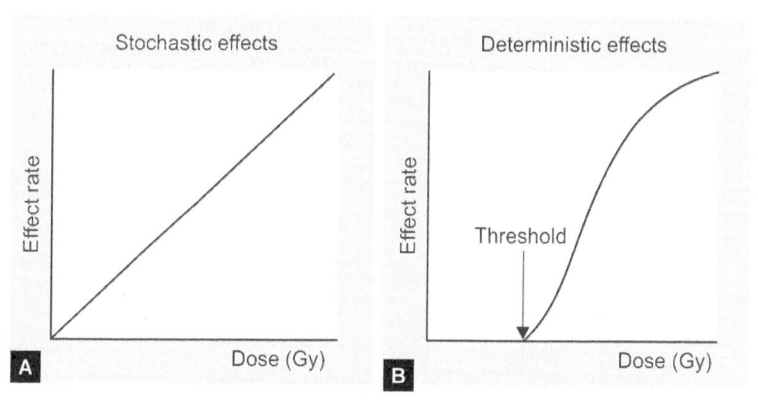

Figs. 10.1A and B: (A) Stochastic and (B) Deterministic effects.

(10–30 years), independent of sex and age. It is likely in diagnostic radiology and nuclear medicine (low-dose radiation < 0.5 Gy). It can be minimized by keeping the radiation exposure *as low as reasonably achievable* (ALARA) and cannot be prevented.

Dose Response Model

Attempts were being made to create a dose-response model for stochastic effect. It is basically a mathematical relation between radiation dose and human response, which includes early and late effects, low and high dose rate, and threshold and non-threshold. The epidemiological data available is only at high doses >100 mGy (**Hiroshima and Nagasaki** atomic bomb blast). The lowest dose where excess cancer has been observed is 100 mSv. What we need in hospital situation is 0–10 mSv, which is not available. Hence, several models were suggested to extend the curve from the high-dose region to low-dose region. This includes hypersensitivity, hormesis, and threshold curves (Fig. 10.2). At present *linear non-threshold* (LNT) model is accepted as dose response for stochastic effects (BEIR-VII REPORT).

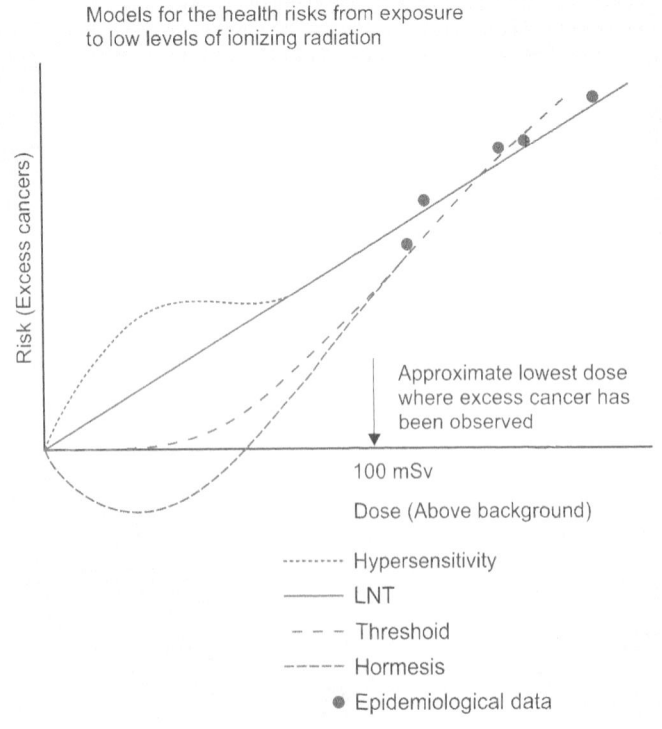

Fig. 10.2: Dose response model.

Radiobiological Basis of Diagnostic X-rays

Diagnostic X-rays are used in about 80% of the medical investigations involving radiation. When X-rays are passed through the patient almost greater than 98% being absorbed and less than 2% is only transmitted, which forms the final radiological image. The radiation dose to the patient depends upon the following factors:
- Patient thickness
- Field size of the X-ray beam
- Source to object distance
- Exposure factors; kVp and mAS
- Use of contrast.

The estimation of radiation dose to each patient is tedious process and hence, general values are recommended (Table 10.1).

The effective dose is the whole body dose that would produce same biological effect as the actual dose from the procedure. The diagnostic X-rays are not penetrating, and are being absorbed much and damage the skin. It may cause skin reddening, hair loss and desquamation in the form of deterministic effects. However, it is unlikely in hospital setup, since our doses are very low. The threshold dose for *skin erythema* is 2 Gy.

The *gonads* are very sensitive to diagnostic X-rays. A dose of 6 Gy is required to create permanent sterility in male and females. Pregnant women can be taken for X-ray, provided there is a clinical warrant. Of course, the risks and benefits must be discussed, before taking the X-rays. Current studies have shown that a radiation exposure of 0.5 Gy may produce *cataract*. Hence, the annual dose limit is reduced from 150 to 20 mSv per year. Use of eye shield may protect the situation of high level exposure.

Diagnostic X-rays has minimal risk towards *thyroid*, except in CT scan of neck. All other examinations only give scattered radiation to thyroid, for which the risk is very minimal. Any diagnostic examination that has a dose less than 100 mSv has no risk to the patient. However, there is no radiological examination that can give the dose 100 mSv.

Chest X-rays can cause *breast* dose, which is not a concern for males, whereas it is a concern for female breast. However, chest X-ray is taken as

Table 10.1: Skin entrance and effective dose for various diagnostic procedures.

Procedure	Skin entrance dose, mGy	Effective dose, mSv
Abdomen	3	1
Chest	0.4	0.1
Head	1	0.1
Pelvis	3	2
Spine	2	1

a PA view, only exit dose is there in the breast. The exit dose is found to be 1% of the skin entrance dose, which is again very low. Thoracic CT scan can offer a dose of 12 mGy to the breast, since CT is uniformly irradiating the body tissue. Hence, chest X-ray is the choice of initial diagnosis.

SYSTEM OF RADIATION PROTECTION

The principle of radiation protection is *justification, optimization*, and *dose limits*. In every X-ray examination we have to justify whether the benefit of using radiation outweighs the risk. If exposure is justified, then it should obey ALARA principle. Such exposures should be within the prescribed dose limits.

Attempts were made to quantify the biological damage arising from the deposition of ionizing radiation in tissue by different types of radiation. The absorber dose ($D_{T,R}$) multiplied by the radiation weighting factor (W_R) gives the *equivalent dose*. The radiation weighting factors for X and γ rays, electrons, protons and alpha particles are 1, 1, 2 and 20, respectively (Table 2.1, Chapter 2). The *effective dose* (H_T) is obtained by multiplying the equivalent dose with tissue weighting factors (W_T), since the tissue sensitivity varies with the radiation type. These doses are expressed in sievert (Sv). The radiation weighting factor for X-rays, gamma rays, and electron is 1. It is 2 and 20 for proton and alpha particles, respectively. The tissue weighting factors are given in Table 10.2. The effective dose is given by the relation:

$$H_T = \Sigma_T W_T \Sigma W_R D_{T,R}$$

Dose Limits

International Commission on Radiological Protection (ICRP) employs the concept *detriment* to specify tissue weighting factors and annual effective dose limits for stochastic effects. The detriment will quantify the overall harm to health from stochastic effects of low-level radiation

Table 10.2: Tissue weighting factors (ICRP-103, 2007).

Tissue	Tissue weighting factor, W_T	ΣW_T
Bone-marrow (red), colon, lung, stomach, breast, remaining tissues*	0.12	0.72
Gonads	0.08	0.08
Bladder, esophagus, liver, thyroid	0.04	0.16
Bone surface, brain, salivary gland, skin	0.01	0.04
Total		1.00

*Adrenals, extrathoracic region, gallbladder, heart, kidneys, lymphatic nodes, muscle, oral mucosa, pancreas, prostate, small intestine, spleen, thymus, uterus/cervix.
(ICRP: International Commission on Radiological Protection)

exposure of different parts of the body. The tissue-specific detriment is determined from the nominal tissue-specific risk coefficient, weighted by the severity of the disease in terms of lethality, impact on quality of life, and years of life lost. Total detriment is the sum of the detriments for separate tissues and organs. The recommended detriment for stochastic effects is 5.7% per Sv, and 4.2% per Sv for whole population and adult workers, respectively.

The dose limits recommended by ICRP-60 (1991) are given in Table 10.3. The whole body effective dose for radiation worker is 20 mSv per year, averaged over consecutive 5 years, to a maximum of 50 mSv in any single year. However, in India, Atomic Energy Regulatory Board (AERB) has fixed the maximum annual limit as 30 mSv for any single year. The corresponding limits for students and public are 6 mSv and 1 mSv per year, respectively. However, in practice, X-ray technologists receive a dose of about 1 mSv, compared to 12 mSv of uranium mine workers.

In this, the public dose is lesser than the radiation marker, since it includes children who receive no benefits from the exposure. It is not the decision or choice of the public. The public are exposed for their entire life time and are not subjected to the selection, supervision, and monitoring. The public are already being exposed to risks in their own occupations.

Table 10.3: Annual dose limit for occupational worker, student/trainee and the public (ICRP-60, 1991).

Exposure condition	Annual dose limit—occupational worker, mSv	Annual dose limit—student/trainee (16–18 years), mSv	Annual dose limit—public, mSv
Whole body effective dose	20*	6	1
Equivalent dose to lens of eye	20†	20†	15
Equivalent dose to skin	500‡	150	50
Equivalent dose to hands and feet	500§	150	50
Effective dose to embryo/fetus	2	—	—

*Averaged over 5 years (100 mSv in 5 years), not exceeding 50 mSv in any single year, whereas AERB annual limit is 30 mSv in any single year.
†Averaged over 5 years (100 mSv in 5 years), not exceeding 50 mSv in any single year (from April 21, 2011).
‡Averaged over areas of no more than any 1 cm^2 regardless of area exposed. The nominal depth is 0.7 mg cm^2.
§Averaged over areas of the skin not exceeding about 100 cm^2.
Note: Sievert (Sv) is the unit used to measure the effective dose in radiation protection. 1 Sv = 1 J/kg. Rem is the special unit of effective dose. 1 mSv = 100 mrem.
(ICRP: International Commission on Radiological Protection)

The ICRP (2011) has reduced the lens of eye dose for occupational workers and students. There are three types of cataracts, namely cortical, posterior subcapsular, and nucleus. Initially eye lens was given 150 mSv (ICRP, 1991) based on the threshold limit of 5 Gy (single dose) and 8 Gy (fractionated) for cataract. But it has no sufficient follow-up to prove the above hypothesis. Ionizing radiation can cause only the first and second types of cataract. ICRP thought that there is a need to reduce the threshold dose for some deterministic effects, which has long manifestation. Hence, ICRP has reduced the threshold dose to 0.5 Gy (both single and fractionated), which is 10 times lesser. As a result, the limit 150 mSv is reduced to 20 mSv for radiation worker for a 5-year period, not exceeding 50 mSv in any calendar year, from April 21, 2011.

The individual dose limits do not apply to patients exposed for the purpose of diagnosis or therapy. Similarly, the occupational dose limits do not apply to medical exposure, natural exposure of radiation, and under conditions resulting from accidents. However, it is our responsibility to include the knowledge of patient dose and the implementation of appropriate dose minimization measures. A radiation worker can be classified as an exposed worker, if he can receive more than 1 mSv per year as a result of his work. Such an exposed worker must be given instruction, personnel monitoring service [thermoluminescent dosimeters (TLD) badge]. If the exposure level is in the range of 1–6 mSv, there is no need for annual medical examination. Medical examination is compulsory, if it is in the range of 6–20 mSv.

METHODS OF RADIATION CONTROL

The three principal methods by which radiation exposures to persons can be minimized are as follows:
○ Time
○ Distance
○ Shielding.

Time

The total dose received by a radiation worker is directly proportional to the total time spent in handling the radiation source. *Lesser is the time spent near the radiation source, lesser will be the radiation dose.* As the time spent in the radiation field increases, the radiation dose received also increases; hence, minimize the time spent in any radiation area. Techniques to minimize time in a radiation field should be recognized or practiced.

All radiation sources do not produce constant exposure rates. Diagnostic X-ray machines typically produce high exposure rates over brief time intervals. For example, chest X-ray produces a skin entrance exposure of 20 mR in less than 1/20 of a second, equivalent to 1,440 R per hour. Hence, radiation exposure can be minimized by not energizing the X-ray tube, when personnel are nearer to the machine.

Nuclear medicine procedure produces lower exposure rate for extended periods of time. The exposure rate at 1 m from a patient injected with 20 mCi of Tc-99m for bone scan is 1 mR per hour. It reduces to 0.5 mR per hour after 2 hours due to decay and urinary excretion. Hence, both the knowledge of exposure rate and how it changes with time are the important elements in reducing personnel exposures.

The time spent near the radiation source can be minimized by understanding the task to be performed and the suitable equipment to complete the task in short interval with safety. Hence, one has to plan the radiation procedure, practice the procedure without radiation and share the essential duties, to reduce radiation exposure. For example, fluoroscopy screening time should be kept short by the use of last frame hold facility, in addition to the use of foot switch.

Worked example 10.1.

A radiographer is performing barium examination under fluoroscopy and the equipment is "ON" for 3 minutes for each examination. The radiation level at the location of the radiographer is 100 mR/h. How many such procedures the radiographer can carry out per week?

The annual equivalent dose limit prescribed for the radiographer is (occupational worker) 20 mSv = 2,000 mrem ≈ 2,000 mR
The permitted weekly dose = 2,000 mR/50 weeks = 40 mR
Exposure rate at the location of radiographer   = 100 mR/h
                                                = (100/60) mR/min
The exposure in each procedure   = (100 mR/60 min) × 3 min
                                                = 5 mR

Hence, the number of procedures
the radiographer can associate within 1 week   = 40 mR/5 mR = 8.

Distance

Radiation intensity (exposure rate) from a point source decreases with distance due to divergence of the beam. It is governed by the *inverse square law*, which states that the exposure rate from a point source of radiation is inversely proportional to the square of the distance. If the exposure rate is X_1 at distance d_1, then the exposure rate X_2 at another distance d_2 is given by

$$X_2 = X_1 \, (d_1/d_2)^2$$

Let 100 mR is the radiation exposure at 1 m for a point source (Fig. 1.3, Chapter 1). The radiation exposure at 2 m is found to be 25 mR by inverse square law. Hence, if distance is doubled, the radiation is reduced by a factor of 4. Keeping larger distance always reduces radiation exposure.

Larger is the distance, lesser will be the radiation dose. This relationship is valid for point sources only, whose dimensions are very small compared to distance under consideration. Thus, the relationship is not valid near (<1 m) a patient injected with radioisotopes, since the exposure rate decreases less rapidly than inverse square law.

In diagnostic radiology at 1 m from a patient, the scattered radiation is about 0.1–0.15% of the intensity of the primary beam. Hence, all personnel should stand as far away as possible during X-ray procedures. Personnel should stand at least 2 m from the X-ray tube and the patient and behind the shielded barrier or out of the room, whenever possible. During the bed X-ray in wards or ICU, nursing personnel need not be panic or run away, it is sufficient to stand 2 m away (adjacent bed level) from the X-ray tube. That ensures effective protection,since the radiation level is almost zero.

Imaging rooms should be designed to maximize the distance between the source and control console. Unshielded radiation sources should never be manipulated by hand. Tongs or other handling devices are used to increase the distance between source and hand.

Worked example 10.2

The exposure rate from a fluoroscopic X-ray machine is 5 R/min at 50 cm. What would be the exposure rates at (i) 40 cm and (ii) 60 cm?

(i) X_1 = 5 R/min, D_1 = 50 cm, D_2 = 40 cm, X_2 = ?
     X_2 = [$X_1 \times (D_1)^2$]/$(D_2)^2$ = [5 R/min × (50 cm)^2]/(40 cm)^2
       = 7.81 R/min

(ii)   X1 = 5 R/min, D1 = 50 cm, D2 = 60 cm, X2 = ?
      X_2 = [5 R/min × (50 cm)^2]/(60 cm)^2
       = 3.47 R/min

Shielding

When maximum distance and minimum time do not ensure an acceptably low radiation dose, an adequate shielding must be provided, so that radiation beam will be sufficiently attenuated. The material that attenuates the radiation exponentially is called shield and the shield will reduce exposure to patients, staff, and the public. If I_0 is the intensity of radiation at a point without shield, and I is the intensity with a shield of thickness t, then $I = I_0 e^{-\mu t}$, where μ is the linear attenuation coefficient of the shielding material. The thickness of the shielding material that reduces the intensity to half is called *half value layer* (HVL) = $\dfrac{0.693}{\mu}$. Hence, larger is the shielding thickness, lesser is the radiation exposure. X- and gamma-rays undergo exponential attenuation in the shielding material. This means that even a large shielding material will not attenuate the

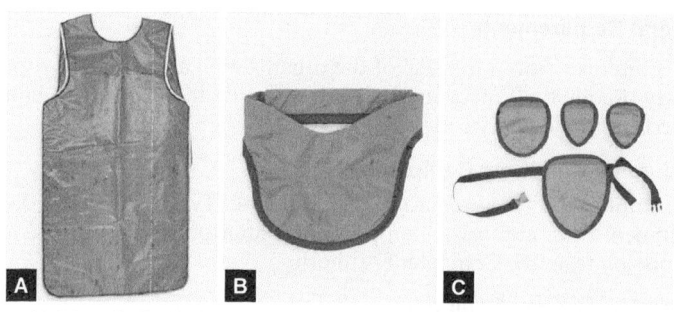

Figs. 10.3A to C: Radiation protection shield: (A) Lead apron; (B) Thyroid shield and (C) Gonad shield in different sizes, to suit the child.

radiation to zero intensity. However, optimal shielding thickness is required to bring down the radiation level below the permissible limit. *Brick* and *concrete* are used as shielding material for construction of X-ray room barriers. *Lead apron* and *thyroid shield* are used for workers safety and gonad shield is recommended for patient protection, especially for children (Figs. 10.3A to C). On the other hand, lead is used as protective material in lead apron, thyroid shield, viewing window, and *gonad shield*. Among time, distance and shielding, distance is the most important method to reduce radiation exposure. Always keep higher distance with the radiation source with sufficient shielding and complete the task with lesser time.

REGULATORY REQUIREMENTS IN THE USE OF X-RAY EQUIPMENT

Atomic Energy Regulatory Board

The Atomic Energy Regulatory Board (AERB), constituted by the Government of India in November 1983, is entrusted with the responsibility of developing and implementing appropriate regulatory measures aimed at ensuring radiation safety in all applications involving ionizing radiations. Before the constitution of AERB, the Division of Radiological Protection of the **Bhabha Atomic Research Centre** (BARC) and the Safety Review Committee of the **Department of Atomic Energy** were responsible for the implementation of radiation safety.

The mission of AERB is to ensure that the use of ionizing radiation and nuclear energy does not cause undue risk to health and environment. Its major objective is to develop and publicize specific codes and guides, which will deal the radiation safety aspects of various applications of ionizing radiations. The AERB implements the safety provisions by the *Atomic Energy (Radiation Protection) Rules-2004*, which provides necessary regulatory infrastructure for effective implementation of radiation protection program in India.

General Requirements
The 'Employer' and 'Licensee' of the organization as defined in Atomic Energy (Radiation Protection) Rules, 2004, shall fulfill the responsibilities prescribed in the safety code.

Procurement of X-ray Equipment
The employer shall procure NOC validated/Type Approved X-ray equipment from authorized suppliers and after obtaining procurement permission from the Competent Authority.

Operation of X-ray Equipment
No diagnostic X-ray equipment shall be operated for patient diagnosis unless License for operation is obtained from the Competent Authority.

Pre-requisites for obtaining License for Operation of X-ray Equipment
X-ray Room Layout and Shielding Requirement

- The room housing X-ray equipment shall have an appropriate area to facilitate easy movement of staff and proper patient positioning. Appropriate structural shielding shall be provided for walls, doors, ceiling and floor of the room housing the X-ray equipment, so that radiation exposures received by workers and the members of the public are kept to the minimum and shall not exceed the respective limits for annual effective doses as per directives issued by the Competent Authority. Appropriate overlap of shielding materials shall be provided at the joints or discontinuities.
- The control console of computed tomography equipment shall be installed in a separate room located outside, but adjoining to computed tomography room and provided with appropriate shielding, direct viewing and oral communication facilities between the operator and the patient. The gantry and couch shall be placed such that it enables the operator to have the complete view of the patient from the control room viewing window.
- Interventional Radiology equipment room shall have an adjoining control room with appropriate facilities for shielding, direct viewing and oral communication.
- In case of room housing radiography equipment, chest stand shall be located in X-ray room such that no significant stray radiation reaches at control console/entrance door/ areas of full time occupancy such that the dose limits to radiation worker and members of public are not exceeded.
- Mobile X-ray equipment, when used as fixed X-ray equipment, shall comply with all the requirements of those of fixed X-ray installation. Movement of mobile X-ray equipment shall be restricted within the institution for which it is registered.

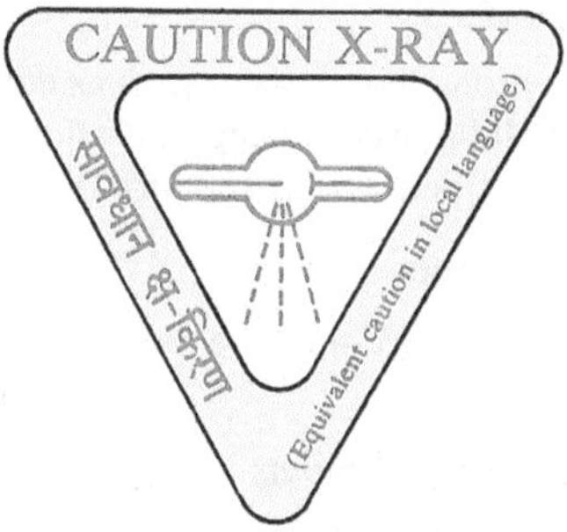

Fig. 10.4: Radiation warning symbol for diagnostic X-rays.

- A permanent radiation warning symbol (Fig. 10.4) and instructions for pregnant/likely to be pregnant women shall be pasted on the entrance door of the X-ray installation, illustrating that the equipment emits x-radiation.
- *Vehicle mounted X-ray equipment*: X-ray equipment installed in a mobile van or vehicle shall be provided with an appropriate shielding enclosure to ensure adequate built-in protection for persons likely to be present in and around the vehicle. Shielding shall be provided around the equipment from all the sides up to height of 2 m from external ground surface. Radiation warning symbol shall be displayed on all sides of the vehicle.

Staffing Requirements

- X-ray installations shall have a radiologist/related medical practitioner/X-ray technologist with adequate knowledge of radiation protection, to operate the X-ray equipment. The employees involved in these activities are considered as radiation workers and shall comply with the duties and responsibilities as prescribed in this safety code. The minimum qualification and training shall be as prescribed by the Competent Authority. All installations having X-ray equipment with fluoroscopy facility, computed tomography and all establishments performing special procedures, shall have the services of a qualified radiologist or related medical practitioner, with adequate knowledge of radiation protection for interpretation and reporting.

Radiological Safety Officer (RSO)

X-ray department shall have a RSO approved by the Competent Authority. The RSO may either be the employer himself/herself or an employee to whom the employer shall delegate the responsibility of ensuring compliance with appropriate radiation safety/regulatory requirements applicable to his X-ray installation. The minimum qualification and training shall be as prescribed by the Competent Authority.

Radiation Protection Devices

Appropriate radiation protection devices such as barrier, apron, goggles, and thyroid shields shall be used during operation of X-ray equipment. These devices shall be verified periodically for their shielding adequacy.

Personnel Monitoring Service

Personnel monitoring services shall be provided to all the radiation workers.

Quality Assurance (QA) Requirements

The end user shall ensure that periodic QA of the equipment is carried out by agencies authorized by the regulatory body.

Servicing

The end user shall ensure that servicing of the X-ray equipment is carried out by agencies authorized by the regulatory body.

Periodic Safety Reports

The user shall submit periodic safety reports in the format and frequency specified by the regulatory body.

Renewal of License

The License accorded by the Competent Authority shall be renewed before its expiry.

Decommissioning of X-ray Equipment

Decommissioning of the X-ray equipment shall be carried out by authorized agencies with prior intimation to the Competent Authority.

RESPONSIBILITIES OF EMPLOYER, LICENSEE, RADIOLOGICAL SAFETY OFFICER (RSO) AND RADIATION WORKERS

General Responsibilities of individuals, who are directly or indirectly associated with the radiation safety of radiation workers, patient and general public are stipulated in Atomic Energy (Radiation Protection) Rules, 2004. The relevant responsibilities with respect to medical diagnostic radiology practice are prescribed in the safety code. All individuals shall comply with their responsibilities.

Responsibilities of Employer

- The ultimate responsibility of ensuring radiation safety in handling the X-ray equipment shall rest with the employer and is the custodian of X-ray equipment in his possession.

- No person under the age of 18 years shall be employed as a worker. No worker under the age of 16 years shall be taken as trainee or employed as an apprentice for radiation work.
- Prior to employment of a worker, obtain the dose records from his former employer, where applicable.
- Every employer shall designate, with the written approval of the Competent Authority, a person having appropriate qualifications as Radiological Safety Officer.
- Employer shall designate those of his employees as classified workers, who are likely to receive an effective dose in excess of three-tenths of the average annual dose limits notified by the Competent Authority and shall forthwith inform those employees that they have been so designated.
- Employer shall provide facilities and equipment to the Licensee, Radiological Safety Officer and other worker(s) to carry out their functions effectively in conformity with the provisions of this safety code, directives and guidelines issued by the Competent Authority from time to time.
- Ensure that provisions of the Atomic Energy (Radiation Protection) Rules 2004 are implemented by the licensee, RSO and radiation workers.
- Health surveillance of classified workers and radiation surveillance of all radiation workers shall be carried out as specified in Atomic Energy (Radiation Protection) Rules, 2004.
- Upon termination of service of worker provide to his new employer on request his dose records.
- Inform the Competent Authority if the licensee and/or the Radiological Safety Officer leave the employment.
- Comply with the terms and conditions of License.

Responsibilities of Licensee

- Establish written procedures and plans for controlling, monitoring and assessment of exposure for ensuring adequate protection of workers, members of the public, environment and patients, wherever applicable.
- Ensure periodic training in radiation safety for radiation workers towards performing their intended task.
- Subject the radiation workers to personnel monitoring and maintain dose records.
- In consultation with the Radiological Safety Officer, investigate any case of exposure in excess of prescribed regulatory limits received by individual workers, implement the follow-up actions, take steps to prevent recurrence of such incidents and promptly inform the Competent Authority of the same. The licensee shall also maintain records of such investigations.

- Arrange for or conduct quality assurance tests of equipment and arrange for preventive maintenance of radiation protection equipment, and monitoring instruments.
- Advise the employer about the modifications in working condition of a pregnant radiation worker.
- Ensure that the workers are familiar with contents of the relevant safety documents issued by the Competent Authority.
- Inform the Competent Authority when he/she leaves the employment.
- Comply with the terms and conditions of License.

Responsibilities of Radiological Safety Officer

The Radiological Safety Officer shall be responsible for advising and assisting the employer and license on safety aspects aimed at ensuring that the provisions of Atomic Energy (Radiation Protection Rules) 2004 are complied with. To this effect, the responsibilities of Radiological Safety Officer are as follows:

- Carry out routine measurements and analysis on radiation safety of the radiation installation and maintain records of the results thereof.
- Investigate any situation that could lead to potential exposures.
- Prepare and make available periodic reports on safety status of the radiation installation to the employer and the licensee for reporting to the Competent Authority.
- Prepare and make available the reports on all hazardous situations along with details of any immediate remedial actions taken to the employer and the licensee for reporting to the Competent Authority.
- Verify the performance of radiation monitoring systems, safety interlocks, protective devices such as lead (equivalent) aprons, and other safety systems such as structural shielding in the radiation installation if any.
- *Advise the employer and the licensee regarding*:
  - Necessary steps that ensure the dose of radiation workers are well within the dose limits prescribed by the competent authority.
  - The good work practices that ensure radiation doses are maintained As Low As Reasonably Achievable (ALARA).
  - Initiation of suitable remedial measures in respect of any situation that could lead to potential exposures.
  - Carrying out periodic QA tests as prescribed by regulatory body.
  - Promptly carrying out servicing and maintenance of the equipment, which can impact radiation safety.
  - Ensuring periodic calibration of monitoring instruments.
  - Modifications in working condition of a pregnant worker.
- Assist the employer and licensee in instructing the workers on hazards of radiation, suitable safety measures and work practices aimed at optimizing exposures.
- Inform the Competent Authority when he leaves the employment.

Radiological Health and Safety

Responsibilities of Operators and Other Radiation Workers

The operators and other radiation workers shall ensure radiation safety while operating the X-ray equipment, as applicable, by adhering to the following:

○ Provide to the employer information about his previous occupations including radiation work, if any.
○ Undergo training provided by the supplier, towards appropriate exposure parameters and dose reduction protocols.
○ Use appropriate exposure parameters for adults and children X-ray examinations.
○ Use protective devices during operation of X-ray equipment.
○ Use personnel monitoring devices appropriately within the facility and monitor dose received.
○ Inform the Radiological Safety Officer and the Licensee of any accident or potentially hazardous situation that may come to his notice.
○ Female workers shall, on becoming aware of her pregnancy, notify the employer, licensee and Radiological Safety Officer in order that her working conditions may be modified if necessary.

Responsibility of Students/Trainees

○ Medical students/trainees shall not operate X-ray equipment except under direct supervision of authorized operating personnel.
○ They shall not receive an effective dose in excess of as stipulated by regulatory body.

Responsibilities of Medical Practitioner

The medical practitioner shall undertake an X-ray examination on the basis of medical requirement. The medical practitioner shall:

○ Be satisfied that the necessary clinical information is not available from radiological examinations already done or from any other medical tests or investigations.
○ Be conscious of the patient dose and for any given examination shall attempt to be in line with international reference levels or those recommended by the regulatory body.
○ Evaluate medical procedures continuously for possible reduction of doses, especially for pediatric procedures.
○ Customize the exposure protocols as per his expectation for optimum image quality for new installations.

Offences and Penalties

Any person who contravenes the provisions of the Atomic Energy (Radiation Protection) Rules, 2004, elaborated in this safety code, or any other terms or conditions of the License/Registration/Certification granted to him/her by the Competent Authority, is punishable under sections 24,

25 and 26 of the Atomic Energy Act, 1962. The punishment may include suspension of license, fine, imprisonment, or both, depending on the severity of the offence.

PERSONNEL MONITORING SYSTEMS

The aim of personnel monitoring program is outlined in Radiation Protection Rules 1971, which was promulgated by the Government of India, under the Atomic Energy Act (1962). The aim is stated as follows:
- Monitor and control individual doses regularly in order to ensure compliance with the stipulated dose limits.
- Report and investigate overexposures and recommend necessary remedial measures urgently.
- Maintain lifetime cumulative dose records of the users of the service.

Hence, the radiation received by all the radiation workers during their work should be regularly monitored and a complete up-to-date record of these doses should be maintained. Personnel monitoring is usually done by employing Film badges or TLD badges or pocket dosimeter. The personnel monitoring devices provide the following:
- Occupational absorbed dose information
- Assurance that dose limits are not exceeded
- Trends in exposure to serve as check on working practice.

In India, countrywide personnel monitoring service is offered by the Radiation Standard and Instrumentation Division, CTCRS building, Anushakti Nagar, Bhabha Atomic Research Centre (BARC), Mumbai - 400 094.

Thermoluminescent Dosimeter

Thermoluminescent dosimeters are used as personnel monitoring devices. It is based on the phenomenon of thermoluminescence, the emission of light when certain materials are heated after radiation exposure. It is used to measure individual doses from X-ray, beta, and gamma radiations. It gives very reliable results, since no fading is observed under extreme climatic conditions. The typical TLD badge consists of a plastic cassette in which a nickel-coated aluminum (Al) card is placed (Fig. 10.5).

Thermoluminescent dosimeter card: The TLD card consists of three $CaSO_4$:Dy-teflon disks of 0.8 mm thickness and 13.2 mm diameter each, which are mechanically clipped over three symmetrical circular holes, each of diameter 12 mm, on a nickel plated aluminum plate (52.5 mm × 29.9 mm × 1 mm). An asymmetric V cut is provided at one end of the card, ensures a fixed orientation of card in the TLD cassette. The card is enclosed by a paper wrapper in which user's personnel data and period of use is written. The thickness of the wrapper (12 mg/cm^2) makes the measurements equivalent to 10 mm depth below the skin surface in the

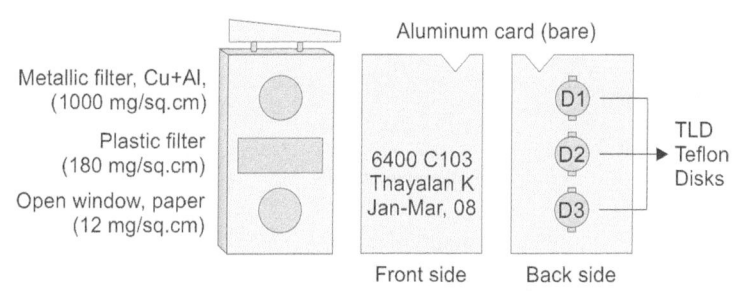

Fig. 10.5: Thermoluminescent dosimeter (TLD) badge, Al cards and its holder with filters.

cassette. To protect the TLD disks from mishandling, the card along with its wrapper is sealed in a thin plastic (polythene) pouch. The pouch also protects the card from radioactive contamination while working with open sources.

Thermoluminescent dosimeter cassette: TLD cassette is made of high impact plastic. There are three filters in the cassette corresponding to each disk namely, Cu + Al, perspex and open. When the TLD card is inserted properly in the cassette, the first disk (D1) is sandwiched between a pair of filter combination of 1 mm Al and 0.9 mm Cu thick (1000 mg/cm^2). The copper filter is nearer to the TLD disk and the Al should face the radiation. The second disk (D2) is sandwiched between a pair of 1.5 mm thick plastic filters (180 mg/cm^2). The third disk (D3) is positioned under a circular open window. A clip attachment affixes the badge to the user's clothing or to the wrist.

The metallic filter is meant for gamma radiation and the perspex is for beta radiation. The filters are mainly used to make the TLD disks energy-independent. When the TLD disk is exposed to radiation, the electrons in the crystal lattice are excited and move from the valence band to conduction band (Fig. 10.6). There they form a trap just below the conduction band. The number of electrons in the trap is proportional to the radiation exposure and thus, it stores the absorbed radiation energy in the crystal lattice.

After radiation exposure the dose measurements are made by using a TLD reader (Fig. 10.7). The reader has heater, photomultiplier tube (PMT), amplifier, and a recorder. The TLD disk is placed in the heater cup or planchet, where it is heated for a reproducible heating cycle. While heating, the electron returns to their ground state with emission of light. This emitted light is measured by the PMT, which converts light into an electrical current (signal). The PMT signal is then amplified and measured by a recorder. The reader is calibrated in terms of mR or mSv, so that one can get direct dose estimation.

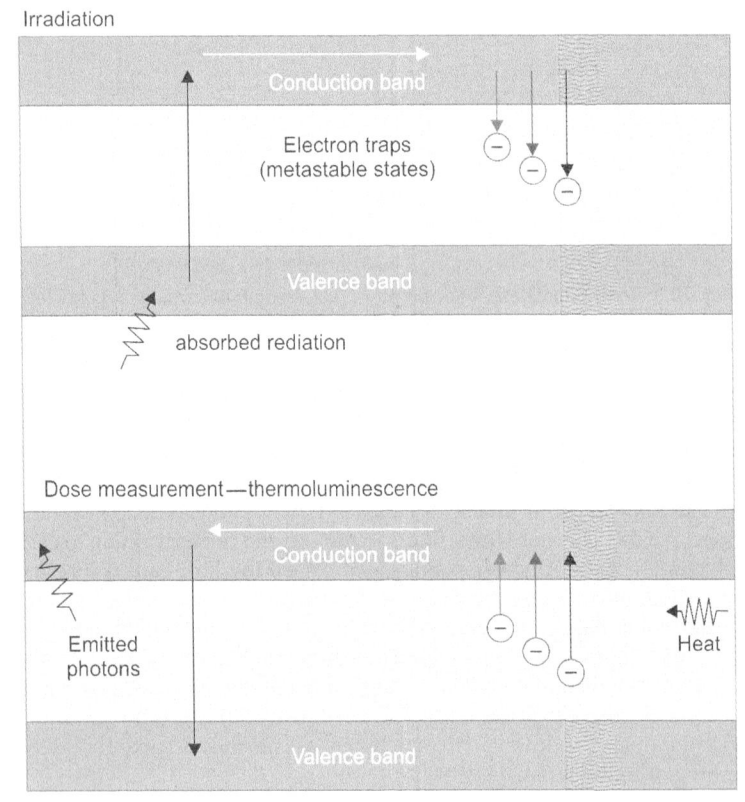

Fig. 10.6: Principle and function of TLD phosphor during irradiation and heating. (*Courtesy*: M/s. Dosilab AG, Switzerland)

Nowadays windows-based computer controlled TLD readers are available (Fig. 10.8). They are capable of analyzing TLD chips, ribbons, powder, disks, pellets, rods, and micro-cubes. They display digital glow curve and temperature profile. They can handle one or more planchets at a time either with manual drawer or computer-controlled drawer function. Programmable annealing oven is also available along with the system. In India, $CaSO_4$:Dy-teflon disks are used in countrywide personnel monitoring.

The disks are reusable after proper annealing, up to 300 times. The annealing process releases the residual energy stored from the earlier exposure. A typical annealing cycle consists of 400°C for 1 hour, followed by 300°C for 3 hours. This badge can cover a wide range of dose from 10 mR to 10,000 R with an accuracy of ±10%.

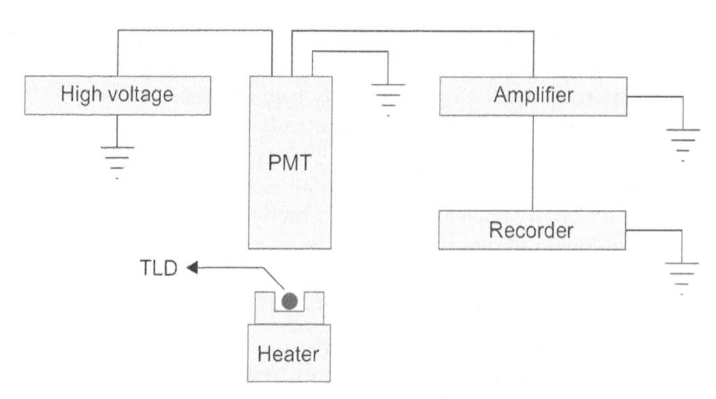

Fig. 10.7: Thermoluminescent dosimeter (TLD) reader.
(PMT: photomultiplier tube)

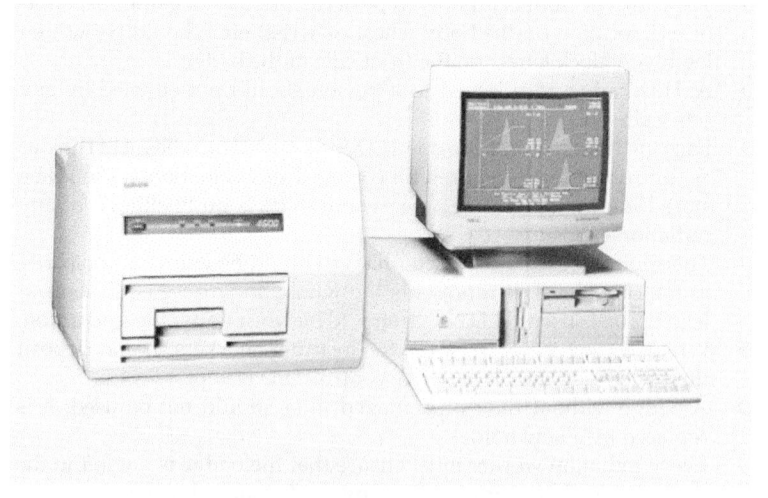

Fig. 10.8: Computer controlled dual TLD reader and workstation.
(*Courtesy*: M/s. Thermo Fisher scientific, USA)

Thermoluminescent dosimeter badges do not provide a permanent record and are available for extremity dosimetry and finger dosimetry (ring). LiF can also be used as TLD phosphor, which has wide dose response over 10 µSv to 1000 Sv. Its effective atomic number is close to that of tissue with an accuracy of ±2%.

Thermoluminescent dosimeter badges are normally worn at the chest level under the lead apron, so that these are expected to receive the maximum radiation exposure. Most of the radiation workers used to wear the badge at the waist level which is not correct. During fluoroscopy, it is preferable for the radiologist to wear at the collar level inside the lead apron to measure the dose to the thyroid and lens of the eye, since most of the body is shielded from the radiation exposure. Pregnant radiation workers should wear a second badge at waist level (under the lead apron) to assess the fetal dose. Additional wrist badge is advised for procedures involving nuclear medicine, brachytherapy source handling, and interventional radiology.

Guidelines for Using Thermoluminescent Dosimeter Badge

- Thermoluminescent dosimeter badges are to be used only by persons directly working in radiation. Administrators, darkroom assistant, sweepers, etc. need not be provided with TLD badges.
- Thermoluminescent dosimeter badge is used to measure the radiation dose. It does not protect the user from the radiation.
- The name, personnel number, type of radiation (X or gamma), period of use, location on the body (chest or wrist) etc., should be written legibly in block letters on the front side of the badge.
- A TLD badge once issued to a person should not be used by any other person.
- Each institution must keep one TLD card loaded in a chest TLD holder as control, which is required for correct dose evaluation. It should be stored in a radiation-free area, where there is no likelihood of any radiation exposure.
- Thermoluminescent dosimeter badge should be worn compulsorily at the chest level. It represents the whole body dose equivalent. If lead apron is used, TLD badge should be worn under the lead apron.
- While leaving the premises of the institute, workers should deposit their badges in the place where control TLD is kept.
- A badge without filter or damaged filter should not be used. It is replaced by a new holder.
- Every radiation worker must ensure that the badge is not left in the radiation field or near hot plates, ovens, furnaces, burners, etc.
- Every new radiation worker has to fill up the personnel data form and should be sent to the BARC accredited agency.
- All the used or unused TLD badges should be returned after every service period (quarterly) in one lot, so as to reach 10th of next month.
- Contact for all correspondence regarding TLD badge service, to the officer in charge, Personnel Dosimetry and Dose Record section, Radiological Physics and Advisory Division, Bhabha Atomic Research Centre, CT, and CRS Building, Anushakti Nagar, Mumbai - 400 094.

Bibliography

1. Arthur G Haus, John E Cullinan. Screen-Film Processing Systems for Medical: A Historical Review. Radiographics, Vol 9, No 6, Monograph: Nov 1989.
2. Chandrakant Manmath Shetty. Computed Radiography Image Artifacts Revisited. AJR. 2011;196:w37-w47.
3. David J Dowsett, et al. The Physics of Diagnostic Imaging, 2nd edition, M/s Hodder Arnold, London, UK, 2006.
4. Donald T Graham, et al. Principles of Radiological Physics, 5th edition, M/s Churchil Livingston E Elsevier, Philadelphia, USA, 2007.
5. James N Johnston, Terri L Fauber. Essentials of Radiographic Physics and Imaging. M/s Elsevier, St Louis, USA, 2016.
6. K Thayalan. Textbook of Radiological Safety. M/s Jaypee Brothers Medical Publishers (P) Ltd, New Delhi, India, 2010.
7. K Thayalan. The Physics of Radiology and Imaging. M/s Jaypee Brothers Medical Publishers (P) Ltd, New Delhi, India, 2014.
8. Kppusamy Thayalan. Basic Radiological Physics, 2nd edition, M/s Jaypee Brothers Medical Publishers (P) Ltd, New Delhi, India, 2017.
9. LJ Cesar, et al. Pictorial review artifacts found in computed radiography. Bri J Radiol. 2001;74:195-202.
10. Radiation Safety in Manufacture. Supply and Use of Medical Diagnostic X-ray Equipment AERB/RF-MED/SC-3 (Rev. 2). Atomic Energy Regulatory Board, Mumbai, India, 2016.
11. Stewart Carlyle Bushong, et al. Radiologic Science for Technologists, 10th edition, M/s Mosby Elsevier, St. Louis, USA, 2013.
12. The Essential Physics of Medical Imaging, 3rd edition, M/s Lippincott Williams & Wilkins, Philadelphia, USA, 2012.
13. Vimal K Sikri. Fundamentals of Dental Radiography, 4th edition, M/s CBS Publishers & Distributers Pvt Ltd, New Delhi, India, 2010.
14. Walter Huda. Review of Radiological Physics, 3rd edition, M/s Wolters Kluwer/Lippincott Williams & Wilkins, Philadelphia, USA, 2010.
15. Walz Flannigan, et al. Pictorial review of digital radiography artifacts. Radiographics. 2018;38:833-46.

Index

Page numbers followed by *f* refer to figure and *t* refer to table

A

Acetic acid 78, 90
Acid 90
Acquisition artifacts 178
Activator 75, 78
Active matrix liquid crystal display 154, 157, 157*f*
Air gap techniques 33
Alternate folder wrapped 50
Aluminium 8
Aluminum chloride 79, 90
American Association of Physicists in Medicine 185
Ammonium thiosulfate 90
    salts 78
Amorphous silicon 134
Analog-digital converter 135
Anti-curl backing and anti-halation layer 46
Antifog agent 76
Aperture diaphragm 29
Aperture size 148
Applied voltage 23, 25
Atomic energy
    radiation protection rules-2004 201
    regulatory board 197, 201
Atomic mass unit 7
Atomic number 7, 8*t*
Atoms 6
Attenuation 33
Auger electrons 9, 22
Automatic film processing 91, 92*t*
Automatic film processor 84, 84*f*
    advantage of 88
    solutions for 89
Automatic X-ray film processing 90*f*
Avogadro's number 4

B

Back scatter 170
Barium 8, 99
    lead sulfate 66
Base 39, 65
Beam restrictor 28, 29*f*
Beryllium 7
Binary digit 123
Binding energy 8, 8*t*
Bite wing film 48
Boric acid 89
Boron 7
Bremsstrahlung process 23
Brightness 97
Buffer 78, 90
Bulb watts 60

C

Calcium 8
    tungstate 20, 52, 66
Carbon-fiber 63
Cassette 56
Cathode-ray tube 94*f*, 154, 155, 155*f*
    devices 187
Cellulose
    nitrate 39
    triacetate 39
Central processing unit 123
Cesium iodide 66
Characteristic curve 51
Charge-coupled devices 19, 134
    applications of 136
    design of 134*f*
Chemical
    memory 40
    pollution 96
Chest radiograph 17*f*, 38*f*, 172*f*, 178*f*
Chlorides 96

Chromium alum 79
Circulation system 84, 86
Cold cathode fluorescent lamp 158, 164
Collimator 28, 29, 30*f*
Commercial computed radiography
 cassette 129*f*
 system 131*f*
Commercial dry laser printers 163
Commercial portable flat panel
 detector 144*f*
Commercial screen-film cassette 65*f*
Communication system 163
Compact disk 154
Compton
 effect 35
 scattering 41
Computed radiography 127, 141, 141*t*, 163, 168
 artifacts 178, 185*f*, 186*f*
 reader 130*f*
  artefact 180*f*, 181*f*
 spectrum 131*f*
 system 130*f*, 184*f*
Computed tomography 149
 scan 93
  resolution 148
Computer 154
 aided diagnosis 182
 basics 123
Concave distortion 187
Cone and cylinder 29
Conversion efficiency 67, 68
Convex distortion 187
Copper 26
Corona wires 161
Crossed grid 31
Crossover 46
Crystal size 77
 and concentration 70
Current 5

D

Darkroom 56
Defective pixel interpolation 159
Deflection coils 156
Densitometer 121, 121*f*
Density 4, 51, 97
Dental film 47, 48*f*
Deoxyribonucleic acid 193
Detective quantum efficiency 68, 146, 150, 151
Detector
 calibration limitation 171
 dose indicators 134
 drops 170
 mishandling artifacts 170, 171, 171f, 172*f*
 offset correction, failure of 171
 systems 140
Deterministic effects 193*f*
Developer concentration 77
Deviation index 168
Diagnostic X-rays
 radiation warning symbol for 203*f*
 radiobiological basis of 195
Diffuse reflection 189
Digital detector systems 125
Digital driving levels 155
Digital image
 format 125
 recording of 161
 viewing 154
Digital imaging and communications in medicine 166
Digital photography 18
Digital radiography 123, 141, 143, 144, 146, 151, 168, 170, 192*t*
 artifacts 170
 optimal image quality in 168
 principle of 137*f*
 resolution 147
 systems 136, 141*t*
Digital video disk 154
Digital-analog 155
Dimensional stability 40
Direct detection flat panel system 137*f*, 140*f*
Direct digital imager 164*f*
Direct exposure film 47
Direct flat panel system 139, 140

Display
  characteristics, evaluation of 187f–189f
  chromaticity 186, 192
  controller 154, 155
  device 154, 155
  noise 186, 191
  processing software 154, 155
  reflection 185, 188
  resolution 186, 191
Distortion 112
Dose response model 194, 194f
Double-door entrance 57
Double-emulsion film 68f
Dry plates 13
Dryer system 88
Dye 70
Dynamic range 153

E

Eastman's box containing gelatine dry plates 14f
Edge-spread function 102
Effective photon energy 25
Electric charge, potential, and current 5
Electromagnetic radiation 9, 10f
  wavelength and photon energy range of 11t
Electromagnetic spectrum 10
Electron 6, 7
  and muons 37
  arrangement of 7, 7t
  interaction with target 21
  volt 9
  with target atoms, interaction of 21f
Electronic data 161
Electronic shutter failure 171
Electrostatic focus 156
Elements 7
Emulsion 40
  absorption 54
  plates 13
Energy 3, 11
Ethylene diamine tetra-acetic acid sodium salt 89

Europium 128f
Exposure index 168
Exposure time 23, 61

F

Factors affecting radiographic quality 97f
Fast scan mode 132
Faults in automatic film processing 117t
Fiberoptic taper 136
Film
  agitation of 78
  contrast 100
  entry system 85, 86f
  handling and storage 54
  material, types of 78
  mottle 107
  packing 45
  processing 74f
  size 45
    and packing 49
  spectral sensitivity of 60
  structure 39
  technology 42
  type 45
Filter 26
  effect of 28f
  spectral transmission 60
Filtration 23, 25
First chest radiograph 16f
Fixer 90
  bath 81
  concentration of 78
  types of 78
Fixing 78
  agent 78, 90
  bath, exhaustion of 78
Flat panel
  display 154
    system 158f
  monitor 158
Flaws in detector calibration artifacts 171f, 173f, 174f
Flexible 40
  film 14

Fluorescent screen 39, 156
Fluoroscopy noise 108
Fluoroscopy resolution 148
Focal spot 24
    blur 110
    size 102, 148
Focus to film distance 33
Focused grid 32
Fuser unit 161

G

Gadolinium 8
Gaussian function and Lambertian distribution 156
Gelatin 42
Geometric distortion 185, 186
Geometric factors 108
Geometric penumbra 109f
Geometric unsharpness 105
Globular grain 44, 45f
Gonad shield 201f
Grain types 44
Green safe light filters 96
Grid
    design and principle 31f
    lines suppression software, failure of 178f
    ratio 31
    types of 31

H

Half value layer 25, 26, 200
Hard disk 154
Hardeners 78, 79, 90
    presence of 78
Heat 4
Helium 7
High latitude film 53f
High tensile strength 40
High-resolution digital imager 164f
Hospital information system 140
Hydrogen atom, atomic structure of 6f
Hydrolysis 42
Hydroquinone 89
Hypertext transfer protocol 167
Hypo retention 78

I

Image
    acquisition technique artifacts 170, 172, 172f, 173f
    compression 182
    display 132
    lag 159
    plate artifacts 179f, 180f
    processing artifact 170, 171, 175, 176f–178f, 182f
    quality 97, 146
    receptor 39
    saturation 170
    sharpness 105
Imaging camera 94, 94f
Imaging device 166
Imaging plate 128, 133f
    cross-section of 129f
    phosphor wear 185
Imaging system
    performance 110
    receiver operating characteristic curve of 111f
    resolution capability of 104f
Indirect detection flat panel system 137, 137f, 140
Ink roller 161
Input devices 124
Intensifying screens 56, 64, 65f
Intensity 26
Interaction with nucleus 21, 22
International Commission on Radiological Protection 196, 197
International Standards Organization 185
Intraoral vertex occlusal radiography 48
Inverse focal spot and calibration 171
Inverse square law 11, 12f
Iodine 8, 99
Ionization 8
Ionizing radiation 8, 193
Isotopes 7

Index

K
Kilo voltage 70
Kinetic energy 3
Kramer's equation 23

L
Laser 161
  camera 95, 95f
  film 49
  printer
    artifact 184f
    functional diagram 162f
Latent image formation 42f
Latitude 53
Lead 8, 96
  apron 201f
  debris near X-ray tube 174f
Length, mass, and time, units of 1
Light, simulation and emission of 131f
Light-emitting diode 121, 158, 164
Line pair 147f
Line spread function 102, 103
Linear attenuation coefficient 34
Liquid contamination 170
Liquid crystal display 158, 158f
Lithium 7
Loading cassette 63
Local area network 167
Low dose rate 193
Low latitude film 53f
Low linear energy transfer 193
Luminance 186
  response 189
  spatial and angular dependence 186, 190

M
Magnesium oxide 66
Magnetic resonance imaging 93, 149
Magnification 108, 148
  factor 108
Mammography film 49
Manual film processing 91, 92, 114t
Manual X-ray film processing, developer and fixer for 82f

Mass 7
  and weight 3
  attenuation coefficient 34
  number 7
Medical X-ray film 39
Metal interface artifacts 171
Modern X-ray tube 24, 24f
Modulation transfer function 102, 104, 148, 191
Mole 4
Molecules 6
Molybdenum 8
Momentum 2
Mono argento-di-thiosulphuric acid 78
Monochromatic emulsions 44
Motion and speed 2
Moving grid 32
Multiformat imaging 93

N
National Electrical Manufacturers Association (Nema)-Dicon Standard 184
Network system 166
Neutrons 6, 7, 37
Noise 70, 106, 146, 149, 153
  correction 159
Non-interleaved film 50
Nucleons 7
Nucleus 6
Nyquist frequency 147

O
Oblique lateral view 48
Occlusal film 48
Ohm's law 6
Opacity and density 119
Operating system software 154
Operator error artefact 183f
Optical
  clarity 40
  density 112
Optimal quality image 111
Orthochromatic emulsions 44

Orthofilm 54
Oscillating grid 32
Output devices 124

P

Pan film 54
Panchromatic emulsions 44
Panoramic view 48
Paper tray 161
Par speed 52
Parallel grid 31
Pass box 61
Pediatric radiography 182f
Penetrometer 113, 119, 119f
Periapical film 48
Periodic safety reports 204
Personnel monitoring service 204, 208
Phantom scattering 148
Phosphates 96
Phosphor 66
　composition and thickness 70
　materials 139
　reader 129
Phosphorescence 11
Photoconductor 126
Photoelectric absorption 41
Photoelectric effect 35
Photo-flo or alcohol 81
Photomultiplier tube 130, 209, 211
Photons 37
Photoreceptor drum 161
Photostimulable phosphor 126, 127
　principle of 128f
Picture archiving and communication system 162, 166, 166f
　use of 123
Pincushion 187
Plasma display panel 158
Point spread function 102, 103f
Polyester 39
Portable flat panel cassette 142
Potassium
　alum 79
　metabisulfite 79
　sulfite 76, 90
Potential energy 3

Power 3
Preservative 76, 78, 79, 90
Pressure 2
Processor quality assurance 93
Proton 6, 7, 37

Q

Quality assurance 113, 166
　requirements 204
　test pattern 187f–189f
Quality control 183
　test 192t
Quantum
　efficiency 153
　mottle 106, 107

R

Radiation 11
　attenuation of 34f
　biological effects of 193
　control, methods of 198
　protection
　　devices 204
　　shield 201f
　　system of 196
　quantities and units 36
　quantum nature of 10
　weighting factors 37t
　with matter, interaction of 33, 35f
Radiography artifacts 118f
Radioisotopes 7
Radiological health and safety 193
Rapid X-ray developer 75
Reader roller damage 185f
Reciprocating grid 32
Reflecting layer 66, 70
Regular X-ray developer 75
Replenishment system 84, 87
Room temperature 70

S

Safe light 46, 60, 61f
Scattered photon 35
Scattered radiation and grid 30
Scintillator 126

Index

Screen
  and film inside cassette, placement of 63*f*
  film
    and computed radiography system 152*f*
    and processor developments 17
    combination, typical function of 68*f*
    contact test 73*f*
    image quality 97
    mottle 106
    radiography 63*f*, 143, 144
    systems 133*f*
    with digital radiography system 143*t*
  function, principle of 67
  handling and care of 72
Secondary factors influencing image quality 98*f*
Secure sockets layer 167
Sensitometer 113, 120, 120*f*
Sensitometry, intensity scale of 119
Short exposure time 111
Signal processing artifacts 178
Signal transmission artifacts 179
Signal-to-noise ratio 151
Silver
  bromide, spectrogram of 41*f*
  from used X-ray films, recovery of 92
Single-coated film 46*f*
Skew distortion 187
Skin entrance 195*t*
Society of Motion Pictures and Television Engineers 184
Sodium 78, 90
  acetate 79
  hydroxide 89
  metabisulfite 79
  sulfite 76, 79
Solid state devices 39
Solution, temperature of 78
Solvent 76, 78, 90
Spatial resolution 70, 102, 146
  test, standard X-ray lead bar phantom for 71*f*

Spectral matching 46
Spectral sensitivity 43*f*, 44
Specular reflection 189
Speed 46, 52, 69
  class 168
Stochastic effects 193*f*
Subatomic particles, mass and charge of 7*t*
Sulfates 96
Sulfuric acid 78, 90
Sulphite 89
Super coat, hardening of 50

T

Tabular grain 44, 45*f*
Target atoms, ionization of 21, 21*f*
Target exposure index 168
Tele-radiology 167
Temperature 77
  and heat 4
  control system 84, 85
Temporal resolution 102
Thermoluminescent dosimeter 198, 208
  badge 209*f*, 212
  card 208
  cassette 209
  reader 211*f*
Thin film transistor 137, 140, 141, 157, 175
  readout process 138*f*
Thyroid shield 201*f*
Time scale sensitometry 119
Time-temperature development 83
Tissue weighting 196*t*
Transmission control protocol 167
Transport system 84
Tube current 23, 27*f*
Tungsten 8
Typical X-ray film box 50*f*

V

Vehicle mounted X-ray equipment 203
Veiling glare 186, 192
Video Electronics Standards Association 185
Virtual private network 167

W

Water system 87
Wavelength 11
Wide area network 167

X

X-ray
    after discovery of 15
    and light field, alignment of 30f
    beam intensity 99f
    discovery of 20
    equipment
        decommissioning of 204
        operation of 202
        procurement of 202
        use of 201
    exposure provides electrons 42f
    film 39
        characteristic curve of 52f
    cross-section 39f
    hanger 64f
    processing 74
    view box for 165f
    images 38
    intensity of 25
    production of 20
    properties of 20
    quality of 25
    room layout and shielding
        requirement 202
    spectra 22
    spectrum consisting
        bremsstrahlung and
        characteristic X-rays 23f

Z

Zinc sulfide 66
Zinc-cadmium sulfide 20